SOUL FUSION HEALING

Integrating Mind, Body, and Soul

MARVIN L. WILKERSON

ISBN   978-1-965360-53-8

Dedication

I want to dedicate this book to several people who have been instrumental in my journey of self-discovery. First, I want to thank my mother, Sally Ann Carrol, who encouraged me to pursue a greater understanding of belief in a Spiritual quest at a young age. To Vicki Green, my first Astrology teacher, for her wisdom and guidance in the realm of an expanded universe. To Robert Kent "Buz" Myers, who taught me about Native American philosophies and Spiritual Astrology. How do we apply and walk the talk, as he used to say?

I am deeply grateful to my wife, Sharon Ann Wilkerson. The love of my life challenged me to become a man and live on a spiritual path, guiding me to my greatest successes. Her support and help in presenting my life's work have been extraordinary and could not have been offered without her. Her Soul has always been my inspiration.

Forward

Sharon Wilkerson

Soul Fusion Healing is a guide for sacred integration. In our journey through life, we can find ourselves experiencing emotional turbulence, physical challenges, and internal longing for inner peace. This book answers the call for a deep understanding of what keeps us in conflict physically, mentally, emotionally, and spiritually.

Marvin draws from ancient wisdom, metaphysical insights, and modern techniques to give you a roadmap for reconnecting with your authentic self. This book lets you grasp the large picture and deeply understand the details necessary for realizing your authentic self. The quotes offer you an opportunity to pause and integrate the information provided into your awareness. Pausing and reflecting along the way is highly beneficial.

As you explore new perspectives on healing and tap into the energy fields that shape your experiences, you will discover your pathway toward transformation. True wellness comes from aligning the mind, body, and soul into a cohesive flow. As you break through your karmic patterns and reprogram your subconscious, you will experience and elevate your spiritual awareness.

As we traverse this modern age, where distraction and disconnection often prevail, Soul Fusion Healing reminds us of our innate capacity to heal from within. Marvin L. Wilkerson has crafted a unique approach, blending indigenous wisdom with contemporary healing modalities, helping individuals reclaim their wholeness and achieve balance.

I have been blessed to observe Marvin's continuous thirst for knowledge and wisdom. Writing this Soul Fusion Healing book is the fusion of thousands of hours of learning on many levels. With heartfelt intention, this book encourages you to heal, awaken, and step into a fuller version of yourself where mind, body, and soul are fused into one cohesive experience.

May this work inspire you to walk your healing path with grace, wisdom, and courage.

Preface

We live in a world that often views the mind, body, and soul as separate entities, compartmentalizing each aspect of our being. Western medicine treats the body as a physical machine, psychology focuses on the mind, and spirituality is relegated to a distant, often misunderstood realm. Yet, throughout my years as a holistic healer, I have realized that true wellness emerges when we integrate these dimensions, unifying our physical, mental, emotional, and spiritual aspects. It is from this understanding that *Soul Fusion Healing* was born.

This book represents my journey to becoming a holistic healer and a lifelong student of the seen and unseen forces shaping our lives. Over the decades, I have studied ancient wisdom, indigenous healing practices, Evolutionary and Spiritual Astrology, and modern modalities such as Hypnotherapy and Neurolinguistic Programming (NLP). These diverse systems have guided me toward one central truth: healing is not a linear process but a fusion—a weaving of all we are into a harmonious whole.

In writing *Soul Fusion Healing*, I aim to offer a comprehensive yet practical guide for anyone seeking to embark on this transformative journey. This book is designed for those who feel disconnected from their authentic self, those who seek healing beyond the physical symptoms, and those ready to deepen their spiritual awareness. Whether you are struggling with long-standing emotional patterns, physical ailments, or spiritual confusion, the tools and insights presented here will help you realign and heal from within.

Each chapter is crafted to guide you through self-discovery and healing, blending ancient wisdom with contemporary practices. Through Evolutionary and Spiritual astrology, you'll uncover karmic patterns and soul lessons. With Hypnotherapy, you'll tap into the subconscious mind, breaking free from limiting beliefs and deep-seated traumas. Neurolinguistic Programming will aid you in rewiring the mind for greater clarity and intention. And most importantly, you'll discover the robust interconnection between your mind, body, and soul, recognizing that healing in one area influences the whole. *Soul Fusion Healing* is a book to read and a journey to experience. It invites you to embrace the fullness of who you are and offers practical steps toward living in alignment with your highest self.

As you begin this journey, remember that healing is both a process and an awakening. It is a dynamic experience that requires patience, compassion, and courage. This book is your companion, offering insights, tools, and support for your unique healing path.

Thank you for choosing to explore this sacred journey of soul fusion. I trust that the wisdom in these pages will help you transform your life from the inside out, awakening the healer within you.

In light and healing,

Marvin L. Wilkerson, CH., M.NLP

Contents

Introduction

"I am the soul. I am light divine. I am divine love. I am divine will. I am fixed design."

– Alice Bailey

Marvin Wilkerson

My Spiritual beliefs were built on the foundations of the Southern Baptist teachings. As I neared my twentieth year, I was challenged to read a book presented by an incredible man. The book was "Think On These Things" by Jiddu Krishnamurti. The book presented arguments for me to think through ideas for myself. I had never thought about questioning the rules and beliefs I was taught. The world of beliefs and understanding opened, and I've never stopped searching for truth since then.

As my journey unfolded, I was introduced to new perspectives from Psychics, Astrologers, Edgar Cayce, and metaphysical ideas. I spent many hours at the Edgar Cayce Foundation studying some of his fourteen thousand readings. My thirst for knowledge has always led to a new search for expanding my spiritual awareness.

In the eighties, past life regression became popular through Brian Weiss and Dick Sutphen. I would practice with family and friends, constantly being amazed. By the early nineties, I became a professional Astrologer. In 2012, I began my hypnosis career, working with clients and applying all I had been studying. Of course, learning progressed into helping those who came to me to realize they could "Think for Themselves" and heal their lives.

The desire for completeness and alignment is crucial in a world of chaos and confusion. This book links old knowledge with our current understandings, guiding you to reclaim your spiritual identity, understand karmic patterns, and reach your fullest potential. I offer this book as a path to reconnect with who you truly are. By combining spiritual Astrology, Hypnotherapy, Neurological Programming, and Shamanic practices, Soul Fusion uses healing tools to empower people to change from within.

The extent of our true power comes from our mind, which is the creator of all. The universe gives us many tools to tap into the power of our mind, as Quantum Physics explains that the whole universe relates to itself. Hence, it is recognized that universal consciousness is perfect in design, and once our mind and body have made that connection, healing becomes automatic.

As Astrologers, we look at the planets as energy and how they affect our understanding of life and human nature, which gives off its unique vibration and energy. The human body is a living energy field composed of energy-producing particles, each in constant motion. Our mind, body, and the Universe have a strong connection. We tend to undermine the fact that we have the power to alter our bodies' vibrations to change our moods, improve our physical health, and help us achieve our goals and intentions. Every energy has a vibration, and as humans, we can alter our vibrations following the energy we're using. Astrology is the language of energy.

Humans and everything in creation constitute atoms, the core of which gives off an energy signature vibrating on different frequencies. Astrology centers on the study of various energies and their interactions of mutual relation. Astrology provides a birth chart that maps out an individual's dynamic and vibrant energy patterns. In astrology, we work with elements and different aspects that reveal the dynamism and intensity of how the energies within the individual interact, allowing us to adjust how we use our energy if needed.

The idea is that our energy suggests, at the fundamental level, that everything in the universe is composed of energy. Energy can manifest in different forms, including physical matter, electromagnetic waves, thoughts, emotions, and spiritual energies. It implies that the universe is interconnected through a web of energetic interactions. With the Age of Aquarius already upon us, today's world represents a mental shift in human consciousness and experience. The power of our mind will dominate over the next 2160 years, the length of an era, with increased mental capabilities, science, technology, travel, and our recognition that the universe is filled with other beings. The Brotherhood of Man will begin the march towards more significant social consideration, freedom, creativity, and personal power, the power to heal our lives. The Brotherhood will extend beyond our planet to encompass our Galactic Family. They have been here for a while, cloaked under the secrecy of those in power. The time has come for full recognition of our Universal family. The excitement will build as we move forward with the transition into the Aquarian Age. And many great minds of this age have already begun communicating through Aquarian principles.

Therefore, before delving deeper into the ambiguous and mind-boggling revelations, I want you to know that my book intends to bring personal experience for healing and discovering Universal methods to enrich people's lives. With the study of energies, the Aquarian Age, the Hermetic principles, Hypnosis, and many psychological and spiritual tools, I aspire to help my audience understand their life's mission and their long-held questions about life and bring out their inner ability to heal themselves. How are we going to do that? This book will answer all your questions. So, let's begin!

Chapter 1:
The Mind: Connecting Us To The Universe

"We are part of this universe; we are in this universe, but perhaps more important than both of those facts is that the universe is in us".

– Neil deGrasse Tyson

Exploring the mind and its connection to the universe delves into the profound relationship between individual consciousness and the greater cosmos. It is rooted in the idea that the mind is not an isolated entity but an interconnected part of a vast, universal consciousness. This concept has been explored through spiritual traditions, metaphysics, psychology, and modern physics.

Exploring the mind's connection to the universe reflects a journey toward understanding human consciousness. Whether through spirituality, psychology, or science, this exploration emphasizes that the mind can transcend its limits and tap into universal wisdom and interconnectedness.

We begin our journey from the birth of everything—nature, born of the cosmic soup. Most of the elements were created over billions of years during the lifetime of multiple stars. Elements in your body heavier than iron went through at least one supernova. Plants weigh more than all other forms of life on Earth. Plants comprise 80% of the planet's biomass, while humans comprise only 0.01%.

More than half the body is not human. Only 43% of the cells in our body are human: bacteria, viruses, fungi, and archaea (single-celled organisms). The elements in the body were made in the stars.

"We are souls dressed up in sacred biochemical garments, and our bodies are the instruments through which our souls play their music."

– Albert Einstein

If we consider genetic material, the human genome consists not only of human DNA but also contains DNA from various microorganisms that inhabit the body. Thus, regarding genetic material, the majority may indeed be non-human.

"The fact is that hundreds of trillions of microbial "invaders" mostly in our gut, are necessary for our survival, and there are ten times more of them than cells in the human body. Because the body cannot survive without its microbes, they are the functional equivalent of any of our other vital organ systems."

– Bruce Lipton, Biology of Belief

Whatever other theories we hold, we must recognize "the healing power of nature." Let us look at how nature itself is connected to all.

"Nature is the physician of diseases."

– Hippocrates

In the 1990s, I spent much time learning about Native American spiritual values. My education came from Sun Bear, a sacred teacher of Chippewa descent, and I learned about Medicine Wheels from his disciples. Honoring nature, animals, and trees is the cornerstone for a spiritual connection and healing. I became deeply enmeshed in the spiritual nature of honoring the earth, sky, the Universe, and all life. This passage says it all:

"People must be in balance and harmony to have a better world. The world is made up of people, along with the rest of creation. It is the people of the earth who are out of balance and who need to right their relationship with the rest of creation."

– Sun Bear

His Medicine Wheel helped me find balance and learn to walk harmoniously with nature. I still use the Medicine Wheel to teach my clients spiritual needs.

"The Divine and Humanity: Between the two lies nature. Consequently, the more humans understand and respect nature, the more we live like the Divine."

– Paracelsus, Swiss physician in the early 1500's

One of the most fun reads of my journey was the book The Hidden Life of Trees, written by a European Forest ranger. The connection trees have with other trees is truly amazing.

Discovering the forest and forest floor, I learned about Mycelium. Mycelium is a network of fine, branching fibers that connect all matter on the earth's floor. Fiber is essential for recycling nutrients in ecosystems and breaking down organic matter. Mycelia is crucial in fungi's lifecycle, serving as the primary nutrient absorption and transport mode.

When conditions are right, mushrooms emerge from the mycelium to release spores, which can then germinate and form new mycelial networks. The force of mushrooms ejects spores at a rate more potent than the gravitational pull of Earth's orbit. Every year, fifty million tons of spores enter the atmosphere, where we all breathe the same atmosphere worldwide, sharing the air, breathing, and connection to the underground.

Here again, we see a connection with nature that transcends trees and vegetation. Nature rises above the ground and moves into the air we breathe, connecting us all.

"A human being experiences himself, his thoughts, and feelings as something separated from the rest, a kind of optical delusion of consciousness. This delusion is a kind of prison, restricting us to our desires and affection for a few persons nearest us. Our task must be to free ourselves from this prison by widening our circle of compassion to embrace all living creatures and the whole of nature in its beauty."

– Albert Einstein

The Summary

The human connection is obvious; nature offers the experience of how life naturally organizes and thrives without human intervention.

The connection between the trees, the vegetation, and the characteristics of animals teaches and shows us universal methods and laws at work. We are teaching a birth, death, and rebirth evolutionary journey. We can receive under our feet wisdom from the forest floor, nature, and the landscape where we live, eat, and breathe. It's healing as our feet connect to the body's organs; we receive natural reflexology by walking barefoot on the ground. Imagine the healing of walking barefoot in the grass, in nature, like we did as children.

"As the underground of nature provides messages of hundreds of miles of roots connections, becoming our greatest spiritual teacher who doesn't need to be brought or sought. It's right where we are."

– Sophie Strand, The Flowering Wand

Connecting Us to the Universe

As proposed by Robert Lanza, MD., and others, the principles of biocentrism promote several vital ideas that challenge traditional views of reality and our place within it. In his book: "The Grand Biocentric Design: How Life Creates Reality," he presents compelling ideas about our connection with the Universe. Here are some of the core principles:

Biocentrism asserts that life is not merely a consequence of physical processes but is fundamental to the universe's existence. It suggests that the universe is structured to allow for the emergence and sustenance of life.

It explains that consciousness plays a central role in shaping reality. Rather than being a causal influence of brain activity, consciousness is an integral aspect of the cosmos, influencing how we perceive and interact with the world.

"There are many planes of "thought" below the ordinary field of outer consciousness— and many planes of "awareness" and "knowing" above that of the ordinary intellectual operations of the average mind. These planes are merely the many degrees in the grand scale of Mind."

- Atkinson, William Walker

Biocentrism emphasizes the subjective nature of experience. It suggests that reality is shaped by the observer's consciousness and perspective, challenging the idea of an objective, observer-independent reality.

"Everything we experience is simply a whirl of information occurring in our heads. Space and time are not actual entities, but rather terms that designate the tools our mind uses to assemble information."

– Robert Lanz

Biocentrism highlights the interconnectedness of all living beings and their environment. It recognizes the relationships and dependencies among organisms, ecosystems, and the larger biosphere.

Quantum theory reveals a fundamental interconnectedness between particles, even across vast distances, through phenomena such as entanglement and non-locality. The notion that particles' behavior can be intimately linked regardless of spatial separation challenges our classical understanding of locality and underscores the interconnected nature of the quantum world.

A concept closely related to biocentrism proposes that the universe is finely tuned to support the existence of life. It suggests that the universe's parameters, such as physical constants and laws, are precisely calibrated to allow for the emergence of intelligent life.

Earth's orbit around the Sun is relatively stable, preventing it from veering too close or too far from the Sun and maintaining the conditions necessary for life. The balance between the Sun's warmth and Earth's distance allows water to exist in liquid form, which is crucial for life as we know it. It's a delicate balance, indeed.

"Time does not exist – we invented it. Time is what the clock says. The distinction between the past, present, and future is only a stubbornly persistent illusion."

– Albert Einstein

Space or time is a linear experience of the conscious mind. Space is another form of our understanding that does not have an independent reality. We carry space and time around with us like turtles with shells. Thus, no absolute self-existing medium exists where physical events occur independently of life.

"Some experiments suggest the past, present, and future are entangled, and decisions you make now may influence events in the past".

– Robert Lanz

The forward motion of time is not a feature of the external world but a projection that arises within us as we tie together the events we are observing.

"Time has no meaning without a relationship to another point. It is a relational concept, one event relative to another. There must be an observer with memory. "

– Robert Lanz

A principle only explains how the mind is unified with matter and the universe. Through modulation of ion dynamics in the brain is the control of the movement of ions occurring across the cell membranes of neurons. These ions play critical roles in neuronal function, including generating electrical signals, transmitting information between neurons, and regulating neuronal excitability.

This modulation is vital for processes such as synaptic transmission, neuronal plasticity, and the integration of sensory information. Dysregulation of ion dynamics can lead to neurological disorders and conditions like epilepsy, Alzheimer's disease, and Parkinson's disease. Therefore, understanding how ion dynamics are modulated in the brain is essential for unraveling the mechanisms underlying brain function and dysfunction.

"When something vibrates, the electrons of the entire universe resonate with it. Everything is connected. The greatest tragedy of human existence is the illusion of separateness."

– Albert Einstein

Biocentrism has ethical and ecological implications. It calls for a reevaluation of humanity's relationship with the natural world. It encourages a shift towards more sustainable and harmonious ways of interacting with the environment, recognizing the intrinsic value of all living beings and, I might add, the Universe.

"In the deepest meditative states, one's mind is not self-contained and bounded within itself but connected to something far larger, indeed infinite."

– Neil Theise, Notes on Complexity

Another concept that fits here is "Divine Thought." Divine thought underscores the idea that there is a transcendent source of wisdom and guidance beyond human perception and understanding limitations. It often serves as a foundation for spiritual growth, self-realization, and pursuing higher truths.

In Eastern traditions such as Hinduism, Buddhism, and Taoism, divine thought may relate to concepts like cosmic consciousness, enlightenment, or the universe's wisdom. Meditation and mindfulness are employed to attune oneself to these higher levels of awareness.

In New Age spirituality and other metaphysical philosophies, divine thought may be seen as the result of aligning with higher vibrations or frequencies of energy. Individuals may seek these insights through channeling, intuitive healing, or connecting with spirit guides.

"The "Divine Thought" does not imply the idea of a Divine thinker. The Universe, not only past, present, and future, but in its totality, is that Thought itself reflected in a secondary or manifest cause."

– H. P. Blavatsky

All is Mind, and the Universe is Mental

As we can see, the earth and the universe are undisputedly interconnected. So, how do humans fit into this equation?

"There's no way to remove the observer from our perceptions of the world. According to quantum physics, the past, like the future, is indefinite and exists only as a spectrum of possibilities."

– Stephen Hawking

"All is Mind" is a fundamental principle of Hermeticism, which dates back to antiquity. This philosophical and esoteric tradition explores the nature of reality, the universe, and the self. This principle is often associated with the first of the Seven Hermetic Principles, the Principle of Mentalism.

It suggests that the universe and everything within it, including physical phenomena, thoughts, emotions, and experiences, originate from and are fundamentally connected to consciousness or the mind. This principle asserts that the underlying reality of the universe is mental or spiritual. It implies that the physical world is a manifestation or creation of the universal mind or divine consciousness. Our thoughts and consciousness play a significant role in shaping our reality.

"There is a thinking stuff from which all things are made. And which, in its original state, permeates, penetrates, and fills the inner space of the Universe. A thought in these substances produces the thing that is imaged by the thought. We can form things in our thoughts and by impressing our thoughts upon formless substance can cause the thing we think about to be created."

— Wallace D. Wattles, American Writer

In philosophical idealism, reality is primarily mental or immaterial. This perspective asserts that the physical world is dependent on or even secondary to the realm of ideas, consciousness, or mind.

"Physical reality begins and ends with the observer. What is observed is real; all other times and places, all other objects and events are products of the imagination and serve only to unite knowledge into a logical whole."

– Robert Lanz

"All is Mind" can also point to the subjective nature of reality, suggesting that our minds shape our perceptions and experiences. This idea highlights the role of perception, interpretation, and consciousness in shaping our understanding of the world.

"The connection between any two events occurs only in the observer's consciousness – he "sees" a connection and describes a "pair" of events, hypothesizing a relationship. This relationship is a concept in the observer's mind: no corollary external event needs to exist in the universe. Unless there's an underlying attractor pattern, nothing can be experienced. Thus, the entire manifest universe is its simultaneous expression and experience of itself."

– Dr. David Hawkins, Power vs. Force

"All is Mind" can also imply that consciousness or the mind plays a central role in the creative process. In this view, individuals' thoughts, intentions, and beliefs influence and shape their experiences, personalities, and world.

"No phenomenon is a real phenomenon until it is an observed phenomenon."

– John Wheeler, Princeton Physicist

In spiritual traditions, "All is Mind" may be interpreted as pointing to the ultimate nature of reality as being spiritual or transcendent. It suggests that underlying the apparent diversity and materiality of the world is a deeper, spiritual reality accessible through the mind or consciousness.

"When you examine the lives of the most influential people who have ever walked among us, you discover one thread that winds through them all. They have been aligned with their spiritual nature and only then with their physical selves. The more I learn of physics, the more I am drawn to metaphysics."

– Albert Einstein

Personal reality is what we think, feel, smell, touch, hear, and intuit. The mind forms an identity from personal experience, becoming one's personality. Your mind is thus conditioned to label, classify, and identify your world.

The Hermetic Principles:

Seven 'Universal Laws or Principles' govern the world: Laws of Mentalism, Correspondence, Vibration, Polarity, Rhythm, Cause and Effect, and Gender. These principles sustain the perfect harmony and order of the world. Let's proceed to learn how all seven Universal Laws fit together.

The seven Hermetic Laws of the Universe were handed down by one termed "The Master of Masters." He was known as Hermes Trismegistus. These laws are linked to all the mysterious, occult wisdom, alchemy, hidden lessons, and Astrology from ancient Greece and Rome.

So, the Hermetic teachings of the Gnostics and Early Christians were lost in Constantine's time. His iron hand smothered philosophy with the blanket of theology, losing to the Christian Church that which was its very essence and spirit.

Studying and connecting with these 'Universal Laws' can profoundly affect your life. They work without your awareness, aligning themselves with your mental state without your input.

The physical world we experience through our senses manifests an underlying mental reality. This mental world is not limited to our human minds. Instead, it refers to a Universal Mind or Collective Consciousness that permeates all existence. Our minds are simply reflections or segments of this more excellent Mind.

Throughout history, word-of-mouth contact has transmitted the seven hermetic principles from one instructor to another. Eventually, at some point in the early 20th century, the teachings were gathered into a book named 'The Kybalion' and written by 'The Three Initiates.' Even in modern times, they continue to be a source of occult wisdom, distinct from any genuine faith but potent.

The Principle of Mentalism

"The All is Mind; the Universe is Mental."

- The Kybalion

According to the principle of mentalism, the cosmos might be considered a form of mental projection. This is like the concept of manifestation, which focuses on the power of your ideas to shape the world you experience.

13

A thought must come before anything else for it to appear. Following this thought, God is thinking, or consciousness and the universe is a manifestation of God's mind, which is called universal consciousness. You and I can harness the power of our minds and manifest our most significant potential.

The Principle of Correspondence

"As above, so below; as below, so above."

~The Kybalion

This is a saying that we have all heard before, but perhaps you were unaware that Hermes was the one who initially came up with it. There is a strong connection between this principle and the first principle of mentalism, which asserts that the things we keep in our minds and ideas will become our reality. The numerous planes of existence, including those with lower and greater vibrational frequencies and the connections between them, are the subject of this explanation.

The Principle of Vibration

"Nothing rests; everything moves; everything vibrates."

~The Kybalion

Yes, the idea of 'vibes' has existed for a long time. Vibration theory says everything has a specific vibration, even spiritual force and physical matter. As we know from basic science, atoms and the world are always moving. Our hearts even send out different vibrations when they beat based on our feelings. When we are 'vibing high,' we block out low-level vibrations.

The Principle of Polarity.

"Everything is dual; everything has poles; everything has its pair of opposites; like and unlike are the same; opposites are identical in nature but different in degree; extremes meet; all truths are but half-truths; all paradoxes may be reconciled."

~The Kybalion

The principle of polarity states that things that seem to be opposites are the same in different ways. One easy way to show this is by using both hot and cold. Cold is just not being hot, and heat and cold are temperature. Spiritual energy and physical matter are both vibrations. Hate and love are both on the same spectrum of feelings. Understanding polarity allows you to 'transmute' your emotions, which are at the heart of alchemy.

The Principle of Rhythm

"Everything flows, out and in; everything has its tides; all things rise and fall; the pendulum swing manifests in everything; the swing to the right is the measure of the swing to the left; rhythm compensates."

~The Kybalion

The fifth principle is linked to the principle of polarity, which is a natural rhythm between two opposites. The tide comes and goes. We breathe in and out. Everything is moving. When we understand this concept, we can appreciate the natural rhythms of our lives and the universe, which allows us to work with them instead of against them.

The Principle of Cause and Effect

"Every cause has its effect; every effect has its cause; everything happens according to law; chance is but a name for law not recognized; there are many planes of causation, but nothing escapes the law."

~The Kybalion

The idea of cause-and-effect links everything together. For every action, there is a reaction. Think about it: Are you the cause? Or do you have an effect? This concept is about awareness of our actions, reactions, and consequences.

The Principle of Responses

"Gender is in everything; everything has its masculine and feminine principles; gender manifests on all planes."

~The Kybalion

The seventh principle states that everything has both male and female qualities. Our wholeness represents both sides. There is masculine and feminine energy not only in the physical but also in the mental and spiritual worlds. For creation to happen, these two forces must come together. When both are balanced, a person can better use all the principles together for the most benefit.

Universal Consciousness

The **Universal Mind** contains all knowledge and wisdom and is the source of all thought and creativity. By tapping into this infinite mind, we can access boundless intelligence, inspiration, and potential.

The principle of "All is Mind" has profound implications:

- It suggests that our thoughts and beliefs shape our reality. By changing our thinking, we can change our lives.

- It points to the power of visualization, affirmation, meditation, and other mental techniques to manifest desires.

- It indicates that we are all connected through the Universal Mind.

- It shows that our brains and bodies are instruments through which Mind operates. We are expressions of this infinite intelligence.

Spiritual development and enlightenment involve aligning our minds with the Universal Mind. Understanding this foundational Hermetic principle provides a mystical yet practical framework for inner personal growth and unlocking our creative potential. By living from this perspective, we can experience life more consciously, empowered, and magically.

Intuition: The Power Behind the Mind

Many people are enamored with the psychic abilities of some people without realizing that all people are born with varying degrees of intuitive awareness. We've all heard about women's intuition. Our intuitive abilities can be expanded with an effort to learn to listen to our intuitive voice. I constantly work to teach people to listen to the still, small voice by paying attention to messages called hunches and feelings. When we get over-emotional, our intuition is blocked. I like to explain metaphorically that emotions are fifteen milliwatts while the intuitive voice is two milliwatts of power.

17

I also like to encourage people to use their voices to ask questions and speak to their Angels, teachers, and guides. We all have them. I want to point out the power of the spoken word.

"In the beginning was the Word, and the Word was with God, and the Word was God."

– John 1:1

Even in a practical way, what comes out of our mouths goes into our ears. This reinforces our subconscious mind, the home of intuition, and the value of faith in oneself.

"Daughter, your faith has made you well; go in peace and be healed of your disease."

– Mark 5:34

Learning to listen to your intuitive voice and what it sounds like and trusting the voice over the ego mind's chatter of evaluating, critical analysis, and judging. How often has your conscious mind been wrong, whereas your hunches and intuition have been correct? Many clients usually recognize the conscious voice as wrong compared to the intuitive voice.

"I think 99 times and find nothing. I stop thinking, swim in silence, and the truth comes to me."

– Albert Einstein

Intuition is a complex cognitive process involving subconscious recognition and interpretation of patterns, cues, and information without relying on conscious reasoning or analysis. It is often described as a "gut feeling" or an inner sense of knowing that guides decision-making and problem-solving.

"There are gaps in understanding that will never be filled by scientists and logicians, gaps that only some forms of metaphysical intuitions could hope to fill."

— Neil Theise, Notes on Complexity

Key Characteristics of Intuition

Intuition operates subconsciously, drawing on a wealth of past experiences, knowledge, and sensory information that may not be consciously accessible. This allows individuals to make quick judgments and decisions based on a rapid assessment of relevant factors.

The subconscious may recognize patterns and associations not immediately apparent to the conscious mind. Intuition can provide insights and guide behavior in complex situations by detecting subtle similarities or discrepancies in information.

Intuition is closely linked to emotional intelligence, as it often involves an intuitive understanding of one's own emotions and the emotions of others. Emotional cues and reactions can be necessary signals that inform intuitive judgments and decisions.

A holistic understanding of a situation or problem helps to synthesize various pieces of information into a cohesive insight. This holistic perspective can be valuable for making decisions in ambiguous or uncertain circumstances.

Intuition draws on implicit knowledge, encompassing unspoken understanding, expertise, and intuition gained through experience. This tacit knowledge base can inform intuitive judgments and guide behavior in familiar or recurring situations.

Spontaneous insights or flashes of inspiration arise without conscious effort. These intuitive hunches can be valuable for problem-solving, creativity, and decision-making, offering novel perspectives and solutions.

Intuition is inherently subjective, as individual differences, personal biases, and cultural factors influence it. What feels intuitive to one person may not necessarily be intuitive to another, highlighting the subjective nature of intuitive judgments.

Intuition is crucial in human cognition and behavior, complementing conscious reasoning and analysis. While intuition is not infallible and can sometimes lead to errors in judgment, it remains an essential adaptive mechanism that helps individuals navigate the complexities of everyday life.

Intuition also plays a significant role in the Hermetic principle of mentalism. We often rely on intuition to gauge the reactions and responses of people we speak with. We can adjust how we communicate with others by observing subtle cues such as body language, facial expressions, and verbal responses. I taught a sales team that we size people up in about five seconds while understanding that people decide to buy from us in about twenty seconds.

Intuition can help us make split-second decisions during work or communication. We may improvise responses based on reactions or adapt to better convey our message or thoughts. This intuitive ability can add an element of spontaneity and authenticity to your thoughts and ideas.

When sharing important information, building rapport with people is a must. We often need a rapport to establish trust and connection with others, which can make the experience more immersive and convincing. Especially those you are trying to help overcome a conflict or communicate a different perspective.

Overall, intuition is a valuable tool for connecting with others on a deeper level. An intuitive idea can come in a flash; the wonderful thing is that it produces a vision of possibility. Once there, it can become a reality.

"What the mind can conceive, the mind can achieve."

– Napoleon Hill

∞

Chapter 2:
Understanding Energy Using Astrology To Unlock Personal Potential

"Everything is energy, and that's all there is to it. Match the frequency of the reality you want, and you cannot help but get that reality. It can be no other way. This is not philosophy. This is physics.

– Albert Einstein

The concept that "All is Energy" aligns closely with various spiritual and metaphysical beliefs, including aspects of Hermeticism and broader philosophical and scientific perspectives. This concept can have profound implications for understanding and working with energy in various modalities.

Energy can manifest in different forms, including physical matter, electromagnetic waves, thoughts, emotions, and spiritual energies. It implies that the universe is interconnected through a web of energetic interactions. Understanding that all is energy can be particularly relevant in healing practices.

Techniques such as acupuncture, acupressure, qigong, and tai chi are all energy medicines that aim to balance energy flow through the body's energy channels. Techniques such as aura cleansing and chakra balancing help remove energetic blockages and restore the free flow of energy throughout the body.

From a metaphysical standpoint, this concept emphasizes recognizing and working with subtle energies, such as chakras, auras, and the flow of life force energy (often referred to as prana or chi). It can be integral to Reiki, energy healing, and meditation. These are just a few examples of the many modalities used for healing energetically.

As a therapist, I use several techniques that combine Astrology, Hypnosis, and Neurolinguistic Programming, or NLP for short, to identify and change limiting beliefs and emotional patterns stored in the subconscious mind. Practitioners access the theta brainwave state to facilitate deep healing and transformation on a subconscious level.

Astrology: A Road Map of Personal Energy

"The starry vault of heaven is in truth the open book of cosmic projection."

\- Carl Jung

The challenge in life is learning to use energy within a given framework—the framework of man's law and Universal laws. Doing so allows one to become a Master of Social and Universal laws, especially natural law, the law of nature.

In most texts and mythologies, Divine forces talk to people through nature. Flowers remind us that we can be artistic, animals have stories to tell, and the world and the universe are just beautiful. As a result, it seems likely that a map showing a part of this connectivity or link can help us align with the whole, which will make us whole.

Following Universal laws brings the ego/personality into the correct perception of who we are, the perception of being a spark of God-consciousness.

"You are gods; you are all sons of the Most High."

- John 8:17

Life is energy manifested in the form of the Universal Consciousness. Humans sometimes use this energy for creative purposes, inspiring our efforts and existence and filling us with divine power. Once the creative endeavor is over, the Universe withdraws, leaving us with a potential feeling of emptiness where identification with ego (pleasure & gain) consciousness comes back in. The ego builds up emotional residues of anger, resentment, guilt, remorse, fear, feelings of lack, obligation, or debt when it does not meet its expectations or live up to its standards.

As a spirit coming into this earth sojourn, it acts and behaves according to inner motivation, intention, and desire, with the scope of the Life Plan as a silent background, the guideline, and the stage for the drama of life. The ego's motives and desires overwhelm the being's plan. The ego judges itself for its actions by putting energy into motion against a hidden standard, perfection, God-consciousness.

– William J. Baldwin, D.D.S., Ph.D.

As a professional astrologer, I use astronomy as a personal energy map. Planets are energy that affects humans as well as nature and the earth. The goal of Astrology has been called the alchemy of the personality. Astrology can reveal how we are using different energies in our lives. A birth chart is unique to each one of us. It helps to find a solution to personal and interpersonal problems to fully actualize one's birth potential.

The immediate purpose of astrology is not to predict events in terms of statistical probability but to bring to confused, eager, often distraught persona a message of order, of form, of the meaning of individual life and individual struggles in the process of self-actualization.

– Dane Rudhyar, Astrology of Personality

Humanistic and Psychological Astrology

Humanistic astrology is a modern approach that empowers individuals and promotes self-awareness, personal growth, and self-actualization.

Here are critical aspects of humanistic astrology:

Self-Exploration: Humanistic astrology encourages individuals to explore their inner selves, motivations, and potential. It seeks to help people better understand their personalities, strengths, weaknesses, and life purposes.

Psychological Insight: This approach strongly emphasizes psychology and understanding human behavior. Astrologers who practice humanistic astrology often integrate psychological principles into their interpretations, helping clients uncover unconscious patterns and motivations.

Self-Actualization: Humanistic astrology aligns with self-actualization, realizing one's full potential and pursuing personal growth and fulfillment. It views the birth chart as a tool for self-discovery and self-improvement.

Focus on the Present and Future: While traditional astrology often examines past influences, and predictive astrology focuses on future events, humanistic astrology is primarily concerned with the present and the individual's capacity to make conscious choices and shape the experience of their future.

Personal Responsibility: Humanistic astrologers stress personal responsibility and the role of the individual in co-creating their life experiences. It promotes the idea that individuals have the power to make choices that align with their highest potential.

Transcending Limitations: Humanistic astrology encourages individuals to transcend limitations, including societal and cultural conditioning. It seeks to free individuals from fixed beliefs and encourages them to explore their unique path to self-realization.

Self-Integration: The birth chart is seen as a map of the psyche, and humanistic astrology helps individuals integrate different aspects of themselves. It explores how to harmonize conflicting energies and achieve more excellent inner balance.

Spiritual Growth: While humanistic astrology primarily focuses on the psychological and self-development aspects, it can also incorporate spiritual growth and exploration. With a bit of open-mindedness, a client's beliefs and values rarely get in the way.

Holistic Perspective: Humanistic astrology takes a holistic approach, considering the interconnectedness of various life areas, including career, relationships, health, and personal development. It helps individuals understand how these areas relate to their overall life purpose.

Therapeutic Use: Some practitioners of humanistic astrology offer Cosmo psychology, using astrology as a therapeutic tool to support individuals in their personal growth and healing processes.

Summary

"Healing in the present moment involves resolving the unfinished business of the past, which continues to influence a person in the present moment. The residual mental, emotional, physical, and spiritual energy of past events contaminates the present experience. Resolving the removal of burdensome energies is the goal of any healing approach. Then a person can live more fully in the present and fulfill more completely the details of the life plan arranged before the present incarnation."

- William J. Baldwin, D.D.S., Ph.D.

Humanistic astrology is a contemporary approach that emphasizes personal growth, self-awareness, and self-actualization. It empowers individuals to actively shape their lives and make choices that align with their soul's chosen path.

Planets are connected to energy centers or chakras within the human body. Each planet is associated with one of these energy centers, and working with planetary energies can help balance and align these energies for spiritual growth and healing.

Astrology and Spiritual coaching can help one recognize that physical, emotional, and spiritual well-being are interconnected energy systems that guide our approach. Balancing and harmonizing these energies can promote healing and overall well-being.

"Astrology has no more useful function than this, to discover the inmost nature of a man and to bring it out into his consciousness, that he may fulfill it according to the law of light."

- Alistair Crowly

Using Astrology as a Tool for Healing

"Astrology is assured of recognition from psychology, without further restrictions, because astrology represents the summation of all the psychological knowledge of antiquity." –

- Carl Jung

Individuals can use astrology to solve their personal and interpersonal problems, especially when fulfilling their full natal potential. Humanistic astrology does not classify planets or aspects as 'good' or 'bad.' It reflects what the individual can become and what he is destined to do if he follows the 'instructions' contained in the pattern of the sky, as seen from the place and at the exact time of birth.

"We are born at a given moment, in a given place, and, like vintage years of wine, we have the qualities of the year and the season in which we are born. Astrology does not lay claim to anything more."

– Carl Jung

Astrology is a language that has the power to reveal the archetype of the whole person. Instead of an empirical science, my view of Astrology is a map describing the soul, its purpose, and its character and personality.

"A child is born on that day and at that hour when the celestial rays are in mathematical harmony with his karma."

— Sri Yukteswar

Everyone is, in an authentic way, the center of the universe. Each has a unique location in space-time, setting him apart from other humans and a unique destiny. This connects him to everyone else because we all share the sky, Sun, Moon, planets, and stars. We are all unique, working towards the same realization, that of the one consciousness that truly connects us all.

Astrology's primary goal is to convey a message of order, form, the significance of human life, and individual problems in the self-actualization process. From this form of life interpretation, Astrology can be used to develop and realize the "Self."

Every one of us has a story about an event that we may easily dismiss because of luck or chance. We are also aware that the more we pay attention to the nuances of life, the more we become aware of incidents of synchronicity leading to experiencing our connection to something more significant.

Chinese philosophy believes in meaningful coincidences, the foundation for medicine, philosophy, and even building theories. Ancient Chinese literature did not ask "what causes what" but "what likes to occur with what." A Good attitude produces a positive outcome, while a lousy attitude produces a negative outcome.

"Friend, do it this way: whatever you do in life, do your best with your heart and mind. And if you do it that way, the Power of the Universe will assist you if your heart and mind are in Unity. One must be responsible when one sits in the Hoop of The People because All of

Creation is related. And the Hurt of one is the hurt of all. And the honor of one is the honor of all. And whatever we do affects everything in the universe. If you do it that way, what is if you truly join your heart and mind as one whatever you ask for, that is the way it is going to be."

- Lakota Instructions for Living passed down from White Buffalo Calf Woman

The art and science of astrology, referred to as a consultation, accomplishes an understanding of nature, symbolisms, archetypes, links, and synchronicities. Astrology can help us better understand our personal and external difficulties and recognize the primary component patterns in our lives.

We are responsible for the attraction, repulsion, adhesion, and cohesion principles in our lives. Astrology helps us understand why and how we choose to use the energies that bring about our experiences.

We cannot escape influences, but we can choose what influences us."

– Isabel M. Hickey, Spiritual Astrologer

We choose our attitude and how we use our creativity. The experience manifests as we think on a conscious and subconscious level, affording us an understanding of what's happening in our lives and why through the astrological map.

You are what you think, having become what you thought."

– Buddha

Astrology and Hypnosis as Tools for Achieving Your Full Potential

A person's astrological chart can tell you a lot about their personality. It shows how and where we use energy and how we have used various energies. Interpretation can evaluate where we need to improve our use of energy. By understanding what we did well and not so well in the past.

We are souls and use an ego structure that helps us see and work with physical reality. Astrology is like a plan that shows a soul's journey. The soul creates personalities to learn and grow through experiences it needs for evolution. A recognition that will eventually show who each person is as a co-creator of their journey.

"What is a soul? According to many spiritual, religious, and metaphysical sources, including the Bhagavad Gita and the Bible, the Soul is an immutable consciousness with its individuality or identity that remains intact from life to life. In each lifetime, the Soul manifests a personality that has a subjective consciousness and unconsciousness."

– Jeffry Wolf Green, Astrologer

Having this map lets you figure out what the soul wants in a particular experience so that you can grow and gain a better understanding of the true self. It also shows the personality any illusions linked to itself for ego and desire reasons.

The map also shows how the journey's activities, environment, route, process, and details align with the soul's goal. The personality can accept or reject the details of the journey to its success or peril. The soul made a perfect plan. As the trip goes on, the personality and ego must discover the accurate perception and perspective that leads to a greater understanding of self. We find fulfillment while submitting our willfulness to the guidance of the soul.

Astrology is the best map to help people see their attachments to false perceptions because energy is pure; how we use it, shape, and mold it can be distorted and painful. Our ego and personality have made up false ideas about needs, desires, and relationships to feel safe, and these ideas can lead to illusions. Therefore, astrology reading is the best way to compare and understand thoughts and beliefs and why people think and feel the way they do, which leads to conflict.

Reality shaped by point of view vs. inner truth causes disagreement and illusion. Once you know what the journey is and what the map shows, you can change your point of view, how you choose to experience life, and what you've manifested. This helps people live in better harmony with who they are and what their soul wants since the soul is the perfect light that leads back to the source.

Areas a Consultation can Reveal

Mind, Will

The conscious mind and the subconscious mind are both identified by astrology. Along with a person's character and ego, a horoscope shows their 'will' and the problems that can arise when their ego or will is too big or too small.

Mentality

We use the word 'mental' to refer to the ways we hurt ourselves with our conscious ego-driven beliefs and those buried deep in our subconscious mind. These patterns comprise many different thoughts, acts, and goals in life.

Family Dynamics and Patterns

Astrology can help one understand how people are imprinted and conditioned by parents, families, friends, teachers, peers, society, and whomever we put on a pedestal. And, of course, the memories made from past lives and experiences.

Programming/conditioning =

"By the time we are 21 yrs. Old we have heard from our family, our teachers, and our peers over 60,000 times, who we are, who they are, and what this world is all about to them."

– Ken Keyes

Past lives

From an Astrology consultation, the way you used energy in the past and the habitual use in the present can become very clear as to why one is creating consistent conflict. When a spirit being comes into life, it acts and behaves according to inner motivations, intentions, and desires. Within the life plan, there is a need to discover misperceptions and misinterpretations of human interactions that lead to false decisions, assumptions, conclusions, and judgments.

Karma

Astrology can give insight into incomplete business from the past to find balance in your life by evaluating your *Dharma* and *karma*. The right way to use past energy patterns can bring unity and wholeness into current life circumstances.

A horoscope encompasses several measurements that can tell you much about your past, present, and future karmic events, actions, and ways of thinking based on the present direction and belief. For example, it can tell you if you're drawn to painful experiences or keep having the same ones. These examples show what we call 'self-undoing,' hidden in the subconscious, which happens when a person either has the wrong mindset or continually responds to life, going against stated desires for happiness.

An astrological reading might help you understand the thoughts that keep coming back to you that lead to recurring draws. A professional interpretation can help people be more realistic in their actions and thoughts, letting them reevaluate better ways to think about, plan, and use energy in their life plans. Most people think it's confirmation of something already inside their mind.

To sum up, astrology can help you make better choices, leading to better situations in the long run.

Astrology & Hypnosis

The only thing that works by talking directly to the subconscious mind is hypnosis. When people are hypnotized, their conscious mind steps aside to let their subconscious mind show them the recorded information that feeds their unconscious actions. The wrong directions can be investigated, watched, and then reprogrammed to skip old journey parts that no longer fit the person's current situation.

My experience in age regression shows that most conflict that continues throughout life was programmed in by age seven. Very few people remember when or how personal conflict was experienced.

Some professional estimates put this number at ninety-five percent of people's issues.

Astrology and hypnosis can be used together to change how false information is processed on both the conscious and subconscious levels. When given different ways to look at an event, it can sometimes lead to an *"aha!"* moment that gives you a new perspective and helps you think clearly. If someone keeps attracting dis-harmony, hypnosis can be used to re-experience the event that promotes the attachment, feel the emotion, and change their point of view by looking at the initial sensitizing event from a more mature position.

This process completely changes your thoughts about an event, allowing you to respond from a new perspective. It brings conscious and subconscious minds together, which can now be called healing. When the mind becomes one, it works more balanced and lets a more significant, more unmistakable voice, the soul, direct your actions.

In the same way, we know that working out is good for us, but we still find ways to avoid it. We are using Hypnosis to remove resistance to doing what is beneficial.

Sometimes, though, the pain is so bad that we must be careful not to run away.

"Before you'll change, something important must be at risk."

– Richard Bach

The hypnotic state makes it possible to create selective thinking and eliminate critical thinking. That's what happens when the person is in hypnosis. When we do this, we let our subconscious mind think about and process our lives, habits, and behaviors in new ways that support conscious choices.

35

Beyond that, when space and time are no longer issues, people can access all the knowledge stored in their subconscious. The mind holds an unimaginable amount of information, and one of those memories is of things that happened in the past that are still affecting us now. People can remember things differently when they think about them again from a different angle. This is because they can revisit a relationship or event from the past. Memory lets you look back on something from a different point of view.

"Pervasive change is only going to happen when you know how to take inventory of a human being. Taking inventory requires knowing how people are creating their realities..."

– Richard Bandler, Discovered NLP

Our families and the way our bodies work support karmic or past events that we must deal with. When people are subconscious, they can change useless ways of thinking and let go of the thoughts that bring those things into their lives. This could be good for your physical and mental health because our bodies store many memories in many places, like muscle tissue, cellular memory, and the inner mind. Being physically aware during Hypnosis motivates the person to take an active role in their healing and re-centers and rearranges the subconscious's attraction to bad memories.

While under hypnosis, you can relive a traumatic event and ask your higher self or the Divine to help you improve your thoughts and replace negative feelings with more positive, divine ones. This is one of the benefits of Hypnosis when it comes to healing.

"Oriental teachers taught that just as there was a sub-consciousness below the ordinary plane of consciousness, so was a super-consciousness above the ordinary plane. From the one emerged the things that had

been deposited there by race inheritance, suggestion, memory, etc., while from the other came things that had never been placed there by either race experience or individual experience but which were superimposed from higher regions of the soul."

– William Atkins

We don't usually ask for things when we're in the analytic frame of mind, even though Angels and Spiritual Guides to help are always around. Astrology can help clarify what we want vs. eliminating a negative perception. (pretending to feel one way when thinking another).

In this case, it might help to know how the subconscious mind thinks about how your body responds to your thoughts. Words are not funny or harmful to the subconscious; they don't hear or respond.

On the other hand, it always pays close attention to our conscious mind and messages and follows them as orders. Further, our body reflects our thoughts, so the subconscious responds to our feelings and emotions.

Using Astrology and Hypnosis together can help you become more in tune with universal laws and energy. Each tool is potent, considering how it could change your life.

"Each patient carries his own doctor inside him. They come to us not knowing that truth. We are at our best when we give the doctor who resides within each patient a chance to go to work."

– Albert Schweitzer.

∿

Chapter 3:
The Aquarian Age

"The Age of Aquarius is the age of excellence in which personal purity shall matter."

- Harbhajan Singh Yogi

The hit song "The Age of Aquarius," from 1969, gushes about the world arriving at the "dawning of the Age of Aquarius." It became a rallying cry for the youth-led cultural revolution for those who envisioned a new age of peace, love, and light beyond the Age of Pisces. Over the last century, we've witnessed a blend of Piscean and Aquarian influences. We are 50 years later, fully experiencing the rapid movement into the Aquarian Age.

An Astrological Age is 2,160 years, measured by Earth and its relationship to the Sun and Cosmos. The transition from one age to another is approximately 100 years. Seeing the events worldwide, we are undoubtedly deep into the beginning of the Age of Aquarius. I want to examine this transition and evolutionary process better.

With its unique transformation, death, and renewal qualities, Pluto leads the way forward, forming a new, more powerful reality with a change in consciousness. Pluto will enter the sign of Aquarius from 2023/2024, spending the next twenty years bringing humanity a new reality and structure. If you resist the change, Pluto will bring events that challenge your status quo. If you say okay to change, the rapid changes will be challenging, but you will gradually accept the new consciousness.

Pluto was discovered in 1930 and brought about the discovery of atomic energy. Its energy represents change and transformation at the atomic level, with one complete cycle lasting two hundred forty-eight years. Transformational change has many elements. The primary elements are death, rebirth, and renewal. The passage of a Pluto contact is a five-year process in a person's life or society—two and a half years of de-evolution and two and a half years of evolution. Hence, the death, rebirth, and renewal cycle. To better understand this powerful energy, let's examine how it affects people individually as it moves into their lives.

In an individual's life, it brings to light ego attachments to experiences where that must be released to evolve into greater selfhood. When Pluto moves over a point in a natal chart, it starts a time of dynamic change that is often unavoidable. This change involves breaking down old beliefs, life structures, and behaviors to allow for something new. It usually forces us to look at our deeper selves, including what's hidden in the subconscious. Famed Astrologer Jeff Green calls it the transformation of the "Soul." This slow process predominantly causes the pain and frustration of letting go of characteristics that no longer serve us. The lessons of Pluto are profound, and pain is the great teacher for lessons we never forget. This de-evolution is needed to achieve the required evolutionary process for our journey.

Pluto moves to a critical point during the initial contact, usually showing the first signs of needed change. The energy can feel strong, bringing up unconscious issues and causing tension as one resists change. Pluto may highlight fears or insecurities, starting to deal with these profound conflicts. As Pluto's effect grows, old and comfortable patterns fall apart.

This time can often see loss or significant changes, such as ending relationships, jobs, or other long-term parts of life that no longer support growth. Emotional release happens, allowing for the expression of what has been hidden. This can be challenging, but it is essential for cleansing and healing. Pluto encourages self-reflection and honest evaluation. In this phase, the focus becomes more inward. People often face their "shadow"—the parts of themselves they hide or do not accept. Confronting these parts takes courage but leads to empowerment, allowing individuals to reclaim parts of themselves and understand their deeper motives. Following the breakdown, the rebirth phase begins. This step involves taking the lessons learned, finding new strengths, and rebuilding life based on solid truths. Individuals typically experience a fresh sense of purpose and clarity, no longer held back by old issues or limiting behaviors.

As Pluto finishes its transit, the person emerges changed. Life is built anew, often with a firmer sense of self and purpose. This time brings new strength and a better understanding of one's true capability, moving forward with more alignment to one's inner truth.

Now, let's examine the societal shifts from Pluto's arrival into a new age, Aquarius. Pluto moved into Aquarius on November 19, 2024, starting a significant change lasting until 2043. This time is expected to bring major societal shifts focusing on new ideas, group progress, and changing old systems.

Pluto's time in Aquarius has often matched significant societal changes. In its last time, from 1777 to 1799, the American and French Revolutions occurred, altering government and personal rights.

These events highlighted democracy, the breakdown of old power (death), and a realignment with Aquarius's love for progress and reform, society's ideals. (rebirth)

Aquarius stands for new ideas and technology. Pluto may boost progress in renewable energy and space travel. This time will create new solutions to global problems, leading to a digital age that lets people access information like never before. This will likely shake up current power systems, encouraging fairer and more spread-out governance. This phase may lead to new governance ideas, focusing on community actions and better civil rights support. With a focus on individuality and group health, society may change its views on relationships, identity, and community. There may be increased acceptance of different lifestyles and diversity, reflecting Aquarius's forward-thinking spirit.

Significant changes could occur in how wealth is shared and how economic systems work, including digital currencies and decentralized finance. This may lead to fairer economic setups and the reconsideration of traditional banks. Though this time offers the chance for good change, it can also bring challenges. Fast tech growth might create ethical questions, privacy issues, and the need to close the digital gap. Social unrest could arise as old systems fight back against change, requiring flexibility and strength from people and communities.

Change is a necessary fact of life. How we cope with change is optional. Our human ego prefers staying with the status quo. Managing your life can allow for these massive adjustments peacefully or with rage and anger. In this book, I intend to give you tools to cope with the inevitable changes gracefully.

Understanding the Piscean Age and Aquarian Age helps us understand the context of the transition we are currently experiencing.

The Age of Pisces is often linked to themes of faith, spirituality, intuition, and sacrifice. At the same time, the Age of Aquarius is intellectually oriented and associated with innovation, technology, humanitarianism, a focus on community, and a higher spiritual association that emanates within us through our intuition.

Pluto, a slow-moving planet with intense, transformative energy, is a catalyst. Its entry into Aquarius heralds a period of significant restructuring and change, primarily scientific, progressive, technological, mental empowerment, humanitarian, and social structures.

The Piscean Age

As each age moves through the zodiac signs, the cultural influences and values of the signs are passed down to future generations. To give you a clearer picture of the Piscean Age, here are some of the most important ideas and themes that are often associated with the Piscean Age:

Dreams and fantasies can cause mental delusions and illusions about individual and collective truths. As such, they produce power struggles with belief systems.

People born under the Pisces sign are known to be idealists, singers, painters, and dancers, but also alcoholics, drug users, therapists, and people with a spiritual calling.

Pisces is the sign that brings the need and drive to become like Christ or another deity. Over 2,000 faiths and ideas have come under this spiritual sign in the last 2100 years. It has also led to wars and fighting for rights, power, and control over others. Leading to false hope that what they believe is true. The most significant fault of the Piscean Age is the belief that truth comes from an external source, be it a preacher, sage, or other diviner.

Positive Responses of the Piscean Age:

Spiritual Awakening: The Piscean Age is linked to becoming more self-aware and searching for incredible truths. Spiritual customs and practices grew during this time, helping people and humanity to develop the human spirit and soul.

Renunciation and Regeneration: The Piscean Age, as well as Pisces, is ruled by the energy of Neptune. As the ruler/energy of Pisces, its presence in consciousness began teaching humanity that giving up, letting go, and surrendering was to be reborn into "Spirit." This would restore us to our original state of being. Awakening to our identity. What Jesus said best, "Ye are all Gods." Every spiritual master has considered this surrendering ego domination to the soul a prelude to mastery. He has given up the inventory of the lower nature, the ego, and the human experience to the higher self. The Soul self cannot infuse the lower animal self until the lower is empty of all that it was, our past judgments and perceptions of experience. "Judge not, and ye shall not be judged." The lesser must be sacrificed for the greater.

Surrendering our identity with the ego does not mean treating the physical world as non-spiritual. It is to balance the absolute with the relative and see the unity of spirit and matter through the single eye of divine consciousness. LIVING AS A SPIRITUAL BEING IN PHYSICAL FORM. This is Pisces and the Piscean Age.

Compassion and Empathy: Pisces is associated with compassion, empathy, and sensitivity. It's believed that during this age, there was a growing emphasis on understanding and empathizing with others, as exemplified by teachings such as "love thy neighbor" in many spiritual traditions.

Sacrifice for a greater good: Pisces's keynote is "serve or suffer," which means sacrificing personal desires and ambition by having empathy for others' needs or a more significant cause, such as voluntarily giving up one's own needs for the sake of others or the greater good.

Artistic and Creative Expression: Pisces is linked to inspiration, creativity, and expression. As people shared their deepest feelings and spiritual thoughts, the Piscean Age has seen significant changes in music, writing, the arts, and other creative fields.

Negative Responses of the Piscean Age:

Spirituality and Religion: The Piscean Age is linked to the rise of significant world faiths like Christianity. People thought organized religion and faith were the main ways to find spirituality and knowledge.

"Every word we speak was taught to us by God's spirit, not human wisdom. ...and he cannot understand them because they are spiritually discerned."

– Corinthians 1 2:13

The primary goal of spiritual work is to transcend external conditioning. The individualism of Aquarius will give confidence to our ability to divine from within our spiritual truths without looking outside ourselves for beliefs. One of my favorite concepts is when Einstein is said to have told a colleague, "Don't tell me something I can look up." Implying intuitive knowledge is what we are looking for.

Redemption and Sacrifice: Unfortunately, these attributes were connected to sin. Redemption and sacrifice are given to outside sources of power and authority figures who decide how one is to be redeemed and what sacrifices are to be made.

This diminished people's power to seek their kingdom inside themselves. Too many looked for guidance from external sources, such as men and those in power, and then became subject to their definitions of their existence and spiritual selves.

In the Aquarian Age, we will be independent and demand to think for ourselves. We will take a stand and defend whatever we believe to be true.

Hierarchical Structures: During the Piscean Age, it was common for faith groups and the government to have various levels of authority. Society was usually defined by hierarchical structures, such as those found in religious institutions and government. The world as we know it now lives in a top-to-bottom hierarchy where prominent individuals hold power over those at the lower levels on the totem pole.

As the Aquarian Age strengthens, supreme power will no longer exist; it will be a universal agreement considering all thoughts. The group mind will be dominant.

Illusions and Deceptions: Pisces has a strong imagination, which can be linked to fantasies, delusions, and self-deception. This leads to a false sense of security and a strong defense.

Fantasy and imagination are best left inside the head unless they fit a goal and you intend to act toward achieving that goal. Imagination is the creation of precise thought forms—substantial mental images in mind—with the ability to use those images to channel energy and release the reality of our true nature into manifestation.

"Imagination rules the world because imagination is the power creating the world"

– Napoleon Bonaparte

As expressions of the supreme being, we, too, have the power to image a world—to create or miscreate; everything in our lives is the visible manifestation of the thought forms we've consciously or unconsciously created.

"Imagination is better than knowledge. For knowledge is limited, while imagination embraces the entire world, stimulating progress, giving birth to evolution."

– Albert Einstein

A misconception occurs due to conditioned thinking when a perceived event evokes an opinion. This produces an ego attachment that elicits a response to an illusion. The individualism and mentalism brought on by the Aquarian Age will help us better use our imagination.

Escapism and Delusion: The sign of Pisces is also linked to escaping reality and falling for false beliefs and fantasy. In its worst forms, the Piscean Age may have seen people try to avoid reality by abusing drugs, living in dream worlds, or denying hard facts.

"We are caught in an inescapable network of mutuality, tied to a single garment of destiny. Whatever affects one directly affects all indirectly."

– Dr. Martin Luther King

It is a great struggle to live up to the expectations of the outer world. If we cannot walk the talk, then we must walk away. In the Aquarian Age, we will be less emotionally dependent on false assumptions.

Dogma and Control in Religion: During the Piscean Age, organized faiths and hierarchical systems became more common. This sometimes led to dogma, intolerance, and control over people's beliefs and actions. This could show up as religious disputes, the targeting of different opinions, or the abuse of power by religious leaders.

Aquarius is much more associated with Transcendentalism, which developed in New England around 1836 in reaction to rationalism. Romanticism, Platonism, and Kantian philosophy influenced this idealistic philosophical and social movement. It taught that divinity pervades all nature and humanity, and its members held progressive views on feminism and communal living. Ralph Waldo Emerson and Henry David Thoreau were central figures.

Transcendentalists believe that society and its institutions—mainly organized religion and political parties—corrupt the purity of the individual. They think people are at their best when truly "self-reliant" and independent.

The transformation of oneself brings about the Aquarian transformation of humanity. To transform oneself requires self-knowledge. One must understand one's values and what and who one is to trust others' truth, values, and understanding. Individualism, Aquarius, cannot be secure or chained to any dogma or belief. One must be aware of personal beliefs and ideals for personal growth. Understanding what you are, without distortion, is the beginning of authenticity and discovering your true self, your God self.

Freedom comes by flushing out the old images and patterns etched in consciousness by the lower nature and freeing yourself from the values of others and judgments of our past.

Victimhood and Martyrdom: When Pisces's selfless nature shows up badly, people or groups can feel like victims or martyrs, unable to change their situation and giving up on improving things.

With Pisces' empathy and emotionalism, individuals may find comfort in adopting a victim mentality due to underlying psychological issues such as low self-esteem, learned helplessness, or a desire for attention or sympathy. Feeling like a victim can provide a sense of identity or purpose for some individuals.

The Aquarian Age is mentalism compared to the Piscean Age of emotionalism. Individuality brings about personal responsibility for the life one has created.

Betrayal and Lies: Lies, betrayal, and secret plans are sometimes linked to Pisces. Some people may have lied, manipulated, or broken trust during the Piscean Age, whether in personal relationships, politics, or other areas of society.

Personal power and selfishness were sometimes taken to extremes during the Piscean Age. Individualism for self-aggrandizement can cause the need to protect position and security. Pisces rules secret enemies in Astrology. But who is the greatest enemy? Why our self, where the subconscious mind has all the values, judgments, and perspectives of the past, which must be repeated or objectified by others to learn the error in our perceptions?

"Education in its true sense should be a tool to expand human perception and consciousness, not produce cogs for the larger machine."

– Sadhguru

When our mind (Aquarius) and heart (Pisces) align, trust and faith lead us into our future of becoming all we can be. When looking at the Aquarian Age, both good and bad responses can be explained by how people and groups adjust to the emotions and values of this astrological age. We are moving from emotional reactions to life toward intellectual responses and group mind.

"If the doors of perception were cleansed, everything would appear to man as it is, infinite."

– William Blake

Positive Responses of the Aquarian Age:

Accepting Change: The Aquarian Age urges people to embrace innovative ideas and changes. People and groups with positive reactions are open to creative ideas, technologies, and ways of life.

The hallmark of Aquarius is about changing. In life, we must change to evolve and grow. The status quo is an inherent human need but leads to stagnation. Aquarian rebellion demands we break with consistency and stagnation. It stands for growth, transformation, and excitement for what's coming.

Collaboration and Unity: In this age, individuals feel linked and responsible for each other. Positive reactions encourage people and groups from diverse backgrounds to work together for the common good and unity. There is a sense of belonging when our creative efforts are aligned with a greater need than our own.

"When there is inner quiet and light, a feeling of oneness, unity, and total freedom. The peace is imperturbable. Actions become effortless, spontaneous, harmonious, and loving in their effect. Our perception of the universe and our relationship to it is shifting. The inner Self prevails."

– Dr. David Hawkins

Humanitarianism: In the Aquarian Age, we are concerned for all: the earth, the environment, and even animals, from the smallest to the largest. We are all connected to all. Isn't it interesting that we can stop to consider a tragedy that's happened thousands of miles away? We can feel the pain.

The Divine and Humanity: Between the two lies nature. The more humans understand and respect nature, the more we live like the Divine within ourselves.

Environmental Consciousness: Since growth and sustainability are essential, positive responses include raising environmental awareness and using eco-friendly methods. We will use new technological advances in the Aquarian Age to solve environmental challenges.

"People are 50% genetics and 50% environment."

– Dr. Manuel Estseller, Scientist

Spiritual Awakening: Higher awareness and spirituality in the Aquarian Age will encourage spiritual growth, mindfulness, and personal change. Using a higher consciousness develops intuition for personal guidance and individual truths.

"Angelic realms are essentially the spiritual manifestation of the Creator in the earth. Their role is to provide an aiding influence, guidance, and even knowledge for individuals in their mental and spiritual development. In one reading, these angelic beings are described as "the laws of the universe."

– Kevin Todeschi, Edgar Cayce on Angels

In the Aquarian Age, people will seek spiritual experiences and awareness more uniquely and variedly by developing techniques and practices for personal growth and healing.

Collective Consciousness: The Aquarian Age will bring a more intelligent and open-minded society. Scientists, technology, and people who help others will get more attention.

This includes a more inclusive understanding of our status in the Universe. We will become aware of other life and sentient beings. We know we are not alone; we are all connected with the entire universe, even on the atomic level. Our knowledge is growing through Quantum Physics to understand this concept.

Innovation and Technology: The Aquarian Age is often seen as a time of significant technological changes and innovative ideas. Modern technologies and scientific advances will significantly affect society as it is now, with even greater applications in the future—far more significant than we can mentally fathom today.

Humanity will continue to advance technologically during this time, leading to significant breakthroughs in various fields such as artificial intelligence, space exploration, renewable energy, healthcare, and communication technologies. Social media will continue to grow with online communities and global networks, easing the exchange of ideas and knowledge.

Equality and Freedom: The Aquarian Age is linked to ideas of freedom and equality for everyone. Society will become more balanced, and individuals will have more freedom in their daily lives.

We are not Alone: Aquarius is also connected to alien life. More people are pointing out unusual experiences and sightings, and dreams about aliens are becoming more prevalent. Recognition of other life could change beliefs about all life and the Universe. It is time we let go of resistance to being open and ready to embrace a larger Universe and other species more advanced than we are. Opportunities are immense.

"Impossible is just a big word thrown around by small men who find it easier to live in the world they've been given than to explore their power to change it. Impossible is not a fact. It's an opinion. Impossible is not a declaration. It's a dare. Impossible is potential. Impossible is temporary. Impossible is nothing."

– Muhammed Ali

Negative Responses to the Aquarian Age

Resistance to Change: Some people and groups may resist the changes of the Aquarius Age by holding on to old ideas, frameworks, and ways of doing things.

Aquarius is the sign of rebellion. What kind of groups could be formed? It is also a sign of duality. How will the masses choose to stay separate from those that resist change?

"Life is a series of natural and spontaneous changes. Don't resist them; that only creates sorrow. Let reality be reality. Let things flow naturally forward in whatever way they like."

– Lao Tzu

Fragmentation and Polarization: The Aquarian Age emphasizes togetherness but can also cause division and polarization through revolution and rebellion. Responses like separation, nationalism, and fights between groups are an old, fearful way of resolving differences.

The Aquarian Age will bring changes and reorganizations in social rules that can cause social unrest and instability. Humanity will always face challenges for evolution.

Technological Overload: With all the new technology that comes with the 21st century, some people may become too dependent on it, which can lead to social isolation, addiction, and a loss of identity.

We can already see this occurring. Our children spend hours on games, phones, and other technologies that distract them from the challenging work of self-realization.

Spiritual Disconnection: Spiritual disconnection, selfishness, and a lack of greater meaning and purpose can be poor reactions to modern life's fast-paced changes and distractions.

The Piscean Age, an astrological age that affects values, attitudes, and beliefs, can be characterized by wars and the idea that knowledge brings power. Money, power, and control were necessary, and purpose was found outside us.

Summary: We are transitioning from 'me' to 'we' as we fully transition into the Age of Aquarius, marked by a global awareness shift and a desire for change. New models are appearing that call for peaceful, fair coexistence. In this era of ideas and inspiration, we are bound to reconnect with nature and let creativity flow.

What is the Age of Aquarius?

The Age of Aquarius is a collective awakening of humanity where blind faith is replaced by self-assured logic and passive acceptance by active creativity. The Aquarian spirit, which promotes unity, collaboration, and truth, urges us to break free from restrictions and embrace our collective power. This time is about tangible change, not just lofty notions. Our abilities will improve with the mental gains made through a more mindful approach to our capabilities. We will use technology to communicate and collaborate on answers, advancing science, medicine, and our understanding of humanity.

This Age is about unleashing humanity's potential and creating a network of mutual understanding and growth, not just individual enlightenment. However, this awakening has its challenges. The Aquarian Age needs responsibility and self-empowerment to navigate the dangers of technological abuse and information overload.

A new level of consciousness will emerge from our challenges, from government to natural disasters to the experience of extraterrestrial beings. Some refer to this as a Trinity of Consciousness, about awareness, a unity beyond duality, and connecting us to the divine and a higher purpose. We will develop a mind beyond three-dimensional reality, viewed as a place of education where souls grow, experience opposites, and become aware of themselves—learning about free will and being responsible, recognizing and overcoming ego-related actions, handling connections, difficulties, and karmic cycles.

Developing a fourth dimension of reality adds intuition and emotional depth. Advancing to a greater Consciousness in the fifth dimension offers unity and unconditional love and recognizes connection among all life, including Mother Earth. Reality is seen as separate and part of a larger universal whole.

Governments will align more with equality and inclusiveness. Natural disasters will teach us how to help others in desperation and need, volunteering with resources and manpower where needed. Extraterrestrials bring not only technology and a higher level of intelligence but also the realization of a Universe of connectedness and oneness.

Conclusion

To begin this astrological era, it's essential to become more aware, flexible, and dedicated to the well-being of everyone and the earth.

We can overcome change and challenge by using our expanded intelligence and consciousness to establish an equal, sustainable, and opportunity-rich society and humanity. The Age of Aquarius is about travel, not a destination. It is a call to recognize our minds' power, expand our consciousness, and work together to create a future representing humanity's boundless potential. Now is the moment to open awareness and work together to set up a world as bright as the Aquarius dawn.

The Goose Story – Teamwork
    By Dr. Robert McNeish 1972

When you see geese flying along in "V" formation, you might consider what science has discovered as to why they fly that way. As each bird flaps its wings, it uplifts the bird immediately following. By flying in a "V" formation, the whole flock adds at least 71 percent greater flying range than if each bird flew independently. People who share a common direction and sense of community can get where they are going more quickly and easily because they are traveling on the thrust of one another. When a goose falls out of formation, it suddenly feels the drag and resistance of trying to go it alone — and quickly gets back into formation to take advantage of the lifting power of the bird in front. If we have as much sense as a goose, we will stay in formation with those headed the same way. When the head goose gets tired, it rotates back in the wing, and another goose flies point. It is sensible to take turns doing demanding jobs, whether with people or geese flying south. Geese honk from behind to encourage those up front to keep up their speed. What messages do we give when we honk from behind? Finally — and this is important — when a goose gets sick or is wounded by a gunshot and falls out of formation, two other geese fall out with that goose and follow it down to lend help and protection. They stay with the fallen goose until it can fly or until it dies, and only then do they launch out on their own or with another formation to catch up with their group. If we have the sense of a goose, we will stand by each other like that.

Welcome to the Age of Aquarius

Chapter 4:
Understanding The Conscious, Unconscious, And Subconscious Mind

"A human experiences himself, his thoughts, and feelings as something separated from the rest, a kind of optical delusion of consciousness. This delusion is a kind of prison, restricting us to our desires and affection for a few persons nearest us. Our task must be to free ourselves from this prison by widening our circle of compassion to embrace all living creatures and the whole of nature in its beauty."

– Albert Einstein

It is essential to distinguish between the conscious mind, our critical analytical mind, and the unconscious, subconscious mind. The latter houses our instincts, intuition, and the Soul's voice and guidance.

When making decisions, which mind do you tend to focus on? Do you rely on your conscious mind to change your habits and make yourself more confident, peaceful, and happier, or do you find the subconscious mind taking the lead?

According to neuroscience, your conscious mind runs the show about 5% of the time and thinks by analyzing, evaluating, judging, critiquing, planning, and short-term memory. The subconscious shapes 95% of our reality using long-term memory, emotions and feelings, habit patterns, relationship patterns, addiction, involuntary bodily functions, creativity, developmental stages, spiritual connection, and intuition.

"Subconscious works faster than the conscious mind and won't be interfered with, yet simple in that it blindly follows a task without considering whether it's what you consciously want or not."

Terence Watts, Fellow of the Royal Society of Medicine and Psychotherapist

Generally, your conscious mind refers to what people use to evaluate moment to moment along with motivation and desire day by day. In contrast, your subconscious mind handles your safety and internal functions, is a record keeper of memories, and has continuous contact with your resources and abilities.

Thus, there are two types of minds we use to make choices. The subconscious mind is impulsive, automatic, and intuitive. The conscious mind, on the other hand, is thoughtful, deliberate, and calculative. It is responsible for executive decision-making, rational thinking, and logic. This part of the mind deals with all conscious activities, i.e., all activities that require deliberate focus, empowering us to make intentional decisions.

The speed at which both works is critical to understanding the difference between the conscious and the subconscious. The conscious mind takes about fifty-five milliseconds to process information while it compartmentalizes and looks for similar information, while the subconscious takes about two milliseconds to respond to information. The conscious mind makes decisions based on a reward system: serotonin-dopamine reward, the chemical cocktail produced in the brain that creates joy, gratification, and happiness for a given experience or response.

This obviously would come into play with all habits. For example, in the beginning, smoking is gratifying because you are one of the gang or feel more mature. Of course, once smoking no longer produces these euphoric feelings, the chemical cocktail and payoff go away, and you are left with a habit that usually reconnects to stress or boredom, which becomes a threat to the subconscious mind. If you are 40, that memory may be from an experience you had at six. Fight, flight, or freeze could have been experienced at 6, but at 40, you have gained experience, knowledge, and maturity, preferring to respond entirely differently. But, of course, this requires hesitation for the conscious mind to determine a chosen, preferred way to respond.

Family and society's accustomed behaviors subconsciously condition our lives. Most of these developmental programs are limiting and disempowering. Though there can be other causes, most self-destructive behavior results from having two minds that do not communicate well. They give us conflicting advice, usually beneath our awareness, and we often choose without thinking.

"The subconscious mind is primarily a repository of stimulus-response tapes derived from instincts and learned experiences. The subconscious mind is fundamentally habitual; it will play the same behavioral responses to life's signals over and over again."

– Bruce Lipton, Biology of Belief

The conscious self can undoubtedly make mistakes, but it's our automatic self that usually causes trouble. Motives and prejudices guide us, and we are unaware of our unique frames of reference that are not in sync with reality, old habits of doing things in a particular way, and feelings we try to deny.

The automatic self directs most of our behavior with spontaneous actions. The conscious self is in charge when we take the time to think about our choices, but it can only focus on one thing at a time. Meanwhile, we make many other decisions, both for good and ill. The automatic self has us quickly grab a cigarette while the conscious self is distracted.

The conscious mind checks facts and corrects our automatic responses when they lead to bad outcomes, but the truth is that it has much less control over our actions than we want to believe. The trick to overcoming bad choices and behaviors is not to strengthen the conscious mind so we can "control" ourselves better. Instead, we change our behaviors to respond more aligned with our choices. It takes time to develop a new action when a trigger or urge brings up the old habit.

"Your beliefs become your thoughts, thoughts become your words, your words become your actions, your actions become your habits, your habits become your values, and your values become your destiny."

– Mahatma Gandhi

When we recognize that the responses and actions are no longer preferred choices or actions, we become aware of the subconscious's automatic response. Then, we can change the subconscious through a repeated positive response to support a conscious choice.

"When the conscious mind knows what's in the subconscious, we'll be enlightened."

– Carl Jung

The conscious mind is the mind which holds our ego, personality, and identity. It can see into the future, review our past, or disconnect from the present moment to solve problems in our heads. In being our creative capacity, the conscious mind holds our wishes, desires, and aspirations for our lives. It is the mind that conjures up our positive thoughts or choices.

How They Work Together

Your Conscious Mind

Our conscious mind communicates with the outside world and our inner self through speech, writing, images, thought, and physical movement. The ability to focus and concentrate are two powerful functions of the conscious mind that the subconscious mind cannot perform. These abilities are crucial in changing our lives.

Our conscious mind is responsible for short-term memory, analysis, thinking, and planning. By focusing your thoughts on positive things, your subconscious mind will deliver the emotions, feelings, and memories you associate with positive thinking. By continuing positive thinking, the subconscious no longer responds automatically to a less preferred response.

On the other hand, if you focus on negative things, your reality will be filled with anxiety, fear, and other negativity. If you want to stay with calming thoughts, you must focus on more rational things so that all the negative feelings or emotions will subside. The conscious mind refers to the part of our mental processing that we know, can think about, and manipulate deliberately.

Here are some of the key features and functions of the conscious mind:

- The conscious mind is directly involved with what we are currently aware of and processing. This includes thoughts, feelings, and perceptions that are the focus of our current attention.

- The part of the mind that manages logical reasoning, decision-making, and problem-solving. It analyzes information, compares, and assesses outcomes to make rational decisions.

- The conscious mind oversees voluntary actions and decisions, such as choosing what to eat for dinner or going for a walk. These are intentional actions.

- Information in our conscious mind includes what is processed in short-term memory. This can be things like remembering a phone number long enough to dial it.

- It plays a crucial role in language processing, enabling us to plan and produce speech, writing, and other forms of communication.

- The ability to focus attention on specific stimuli or thoughts and to switch attention between different tasks is a function of the conscious mind.

While incredibly powerful and critical for complex, deliberate tasks, the conscious mind is limited in how much information it can manage simultaneously. It relies heavily on the subconscious and unconscious parts of the mind to process vast amounts of information automatically and inform conscious thought and decision-making processes. This relationship is crucial in holistic and integrative approaches to personal development.

The Subconscious Mind

The subconscious mind is the mastermind producing most of our current reality. It holds onto the beliefs and behaviors ingrained in us during our formative years. It is a vast collection of acquired patterns and beliefs that can operate independently of our conscious awareness. The subconscious mind seems like an autopilot system that strongly impacts our lives.

Our experiences are influenced by the ideas stored in our subconscious. Negative thoughts can impact our overall well-being and longevity. On the other hand, embracing positive beliefs can significantly impact our health and longevity. Like how our conditioning and programming use self-talk that can limit or encourage us, our subconscious beliefs influence our experiences.

We must recognize our negative subconscious patterns and learn to change them through strategies like positive self-talk or mindfulness activities. This aligns with epigenetics, which suggests that environmental factors like thoughts, emotions, and experiences can impact gene expression during growth. Once we understand this connection more deeply, we can use our conscious thoughts and positive reinforcement to influence the programming stored in our subconscious. This, in turn, can result in better health and overall well-being.

Our subconscious mind holds tremendous power, preserving the ingrained thoughts and habits formed during our early years and past life experiences. These beliefs have produced perceptions and perspectives from those experiences. These subconscious programs, formed by our beliefs, can significantly influence our health and well-being. By understanding the connection between our conscious and subconscious minds, we can use conscious thinking and positive reinforcement to influence the stored programs in our subconscious minds, leading to enhanced health and well-being.

The subconscious mind is a fascinating and integral part of our overall psyche. It acts as a bridge between the conscious mind and the unconscious mind. It operates below conscious awareness, influencing many behaviors, decisions, and emotions.

Here is a more detailed look at the characteristics and functions of the subconscious mind:

- The subconscious mind manages automated breathing, digestion, heartbeat, and other processes. These are vital life functions that do not require our conscious attention.

- It is the storehouse of all our learned behaviors and automatic patterns. For instance, once you learn how to ride a bike, the skill is stored in your subconscious. You can then ride a bike again without consciously thinking about each motion.

- The subconscious is closely tied to our emotions. While we might feel emotions in our conscious mind, the associations and reactions that trigger these emotions often reside in the subconscious. This part of the mind processes emotional information and can govern emotional responses based on past experiences.

- The subconscious mind retains memories and past experiences, serving as a vast repository of all the events and learning that shape our behavior and beliefs. This includes not only explicit memories but also implicit knowledge like acquired skills.

- The subconscious mind thinks in symbols and metaphors, which is why dreams are often symbolic. It communicates with the conscious mind through feelings, images, and dreams, usually revealing deeper truths through illogical and non-linear narratives.

- It dramatically influences our conscious thoughts and actions, even though we might not know it. Many impulses and ideas "bubble up" from the subconscious, affecting our conscious decisions in ways we might not fully recognize.

- The subconscious learns through association, imitation, and mimicry.

The subconscious mind can be programmed and reprogrammed through repeated thoughts, affirmations, visualizations, and other techniques. This ability is beneficial in therapeutic settings, where it helps individuals change limiting beliefs and destructive behavior patterns.

Practices such as hypnotherapy, meditation, and certain spiritual rituals aim to engage the subconscious and facilitate more profound personal growth and healing by aligning subconscious patterns with conscious goals and healthier frameworks.

The Unconscious Mind

The concept of the unconscious, particularly in psychological and philosophical contexts, is abstract rather than physical. It is not located in a specific body part like an organ but pertains to mental processes and functions.

"The greatest impediments to changes in our traditional roles seem to lie not in the visible world of conscious intent, but in the murky realm of the unconscious mind."

– Augustus Y. Napier

In psychological terms, especially in the frameworks established by figures such as Sigmund Freud and Carl Jung, the unconscious is a reservoir of feelings, thoughts, urges, and memories outside our conscious awareness. Freud depicted the unconscious as a part of the mind that influences our behavior and experiences, even though we are unaware of these underlying influences.

"Man's task is to become conscious of the contents that press upward from the unconscious."

- Carl Jung

In terms of brain structure, while no one part of the brain can be pinpointed as the "location" of the unconscious, studies often associate it with various automatic processes in the lower-level brain regions, such as the limbic system, which handles emotions and memories, and the basal ganglia, which play a role in habit formation and procedural learning.

The unconscious might also be considered a field that transcends the individual, connecting broader spiritual or cosmic energies and patterns that influence the personal psyche and behaviors. This perspective aligns with more holistic and integrative views in certain spiritual traditions and modern psychological theories, which consider the interconnectedness of all things, including the mind's deeper workings.

"Our life is composed greatly of dreams, from the unconscious, and they must be brought into connection with action. They must be woven together."

– Anais Nin

I also contend that family and ancestors program the unconscious. This programming relates to our feelings, emotions, inhibitions, security, and self-image, among other things. Family is our foundation in life. At some point in growth and maturity, family beliefs challenge us to change problematic beliefs to articulate our authentic selves by choice.

"The collective unconscious consists of the sum of the instincts and their correlates, the archetypes. Just as everybody possesses instincts, so he also possesses a stock of archetypal images."

– Carl Jung

The unconscious mind is a profound and complex psyche component, operating below conscious awareness. It encompasses mental processes inaccessible to our conscious mind but significantly influences our behaviors, decisions, and feelings.

Here is an exploration of its essential characteristics and functions:

- The unconscious mind harbors our most primitive drives and instincts, such as those related to survival, aggression, and sexuality, which are inherited and operate independently of our conscious control.

- It contains memories and emotions intentionally or unintentionally repressed to protect the conscious mind. These can include traumatic experiences or painful memories that are too difficult for the conscious mind to manage.

- Like the subconscious, the unconscious mind processes information symbolically. This is evident in dreams and tongue slips, which can reveal more profound truths and unconscious desires or thoughts.

- The unconscious mind employs a variety of defense mechanisms, such as repression, denial, projection, and rationalization, to cope with anxiety and protect the self from psychological harm.

- Over time, skills and behaviors can become so practiced that they become unconscious, such as driving a car on a familiar route where you might have reached your destination without conscious recall of the drive.

- The unconscious mind profoundly impacts our personality, influencing our thoughts, feelings, and behavior. It shapes our reactions and interactions with the world, often based on past experiences we may not recall consciously.

- Communication with the unconscious mind is essential in psychoanalytic and psychotherapeutic practices. Techniques such as dream interpretation, free association, and the analysis of tongue slips are used to explore and understand the unconscious mind.

Exploring the unconscious can reveal the underlying causes of behavioral and emotional issues, facilitating a deeper understanding of oneself and promoting profound personal change. This exploration can be particularly relevant in practices integrating all aspects of the psyche for holistic healing.

The interaction between the conscious, unconscious, and subconscious mind shapes our perceptions, emotions, and behaviors. The unconscious and subconscious minds communicate with the conscious mind through feelings, emotions, imagination, sensations, and dreams. Much of this communication is seen as intuition or gut feelings guiding conscious decisions.

Most of our behaviors and decisions are influenced by the content and processes of the unconscious mind. For example, a trauma stored in the unconscious might affect how one reacts to similar situations without consciously understanding why.

"We shall probably get nearest to the truth if we think of the conscious and personal psyche as resting upon the broad basis of an inherited and universal psychic disposition which is as such unconscious, and that our psyche bears the same relation to the collective psyche as the individual to society."

– Carl Jung

Information from your daily experiences gets processed in various stages. From immediate and conscious awareness, it moves to the subconscious, where it can be quickly recalled. Eventually, more profound emotional experiences may sink into the unconscious, influencing long-term behaviors and predispositions.

Brainwaves And Consciousness

The human mind is genuinely captivating and operates on multiple levels simultaneously. By studying the different patterns of brainwaves, we can gain valuable insights into the workings of the conscious and subconscious mind and how they work together to shape our experiences.

When we are awake and alert, our conscious mind operates in '*beta waves,*' the primary waves dominating our thoughts. Focus, a sharp mind, and finding solutions are all part of this area. This is where we analyze information, make decisions, and navigate the world beyond ourselves. Engaging in ongoing beta activity is crucial for our daily routines. However, it can also lead to feelings of concern and unease, making relaxing challenging.

'*Alpha waves*' serve as a connection between the conscious and subconscious mind. A calmer and more reflective state can arise from the beta state's inclination to engage in analytical conversation, which

71

is subdued in this context. When you are in the alpha phase, daydreaming becomes easier, creativity flourishes, and visualization exercises are more effective. Now, we can tap into the vast reservoir of knowledge and memories in our subconscious. Imagine alpha as a rich soil where we can sow the seeds of uplifting thoughts and aspirations, molding our deep-seated beliefs and impacting the experiences ahead.

When we are exposed to *'theta waves,'* we can tap into deeper levels of consciousness. The theta state of consciousness is often linked to meditation, hypnosis, and profound creative breakthroughs. This state allows us to tap into a more profound sense of intuition and spiritual awareness. It is also when those moments of inspiration strike us with sudden clarity. Theta can be a gateway to unlock suppressed memories and emotions, potentially leading to healing. Reflecting on our previous encounters and moving ahead with a better understanding and more muscular emotional strength can be valuable for personal development. In this way, we can continue to progress with a greater sense of emotional stability.

Delta waves are fascinating brainwaves associated with deep sleep and dreamless slumber. Research is ongoing on delta waves and their potential connection to non-physical levels of consciousness. As you enter this space, you'll discover a profound sense of healing, renewal, and revitalization. The delta state is crucial for improving our physical and mental well-being, even though we may not be consciously aware of what occurs during this state.

Gamma brain waves are the fastest brainwave frequency, with oscillations ranging from 30 to 100 Hz, though 40 Hz is typical. They are associated with forming ideas, language, memory processing, and several types of learning. Gamma waves play a significant role in sensory processing and are thought to coordinate information from various parts of the brain.

Critical characteristics of gamma brain waves include:

- Gamma waves are linked to improved memory formation and cognitive processing. Promoting neural synchrony can enhance the brain's ability to integrate information, potentially aiding therapeutic practices.

- Higher levels of gamma activity have been associated with positive emotional states and resilience. This can be particularly beneficial in healing practices, as emotional well-being is crucial for overall health.

- Many forms of meditation, especially those focusing on deep concentration or transcendental experiences, can increase gamma wave activity. This has been linked to deep relaxation, healing, and improved focus and clarity.

- Some studies suggest that gamma wave entrainment may help reduce pain perception. Techniques that stimulate gamma waves could benefit individuals dealing with chronic pain or recovery from injury.

- Gamma waves have been reported in states of peak spiritual experiences or transcendental states. These can foster a sense of connection and purpose, which is essential in various healing modalities.

- Gamma waves are involved in processes related to neuroplasticity, the brain's ability to reorganize itself. This adaptability can be harnessed in therapeutic contexts to support healing from trauma or neurological conditions.

Meditative and mindfulness practices enhance gamma wave activity, which correlates with greater mental clarity, enhanced focus, and improved cognitive functioning. This aligns with spiritual practices that harmonize the body, mind, and spirit, often achieving heightened awareness and consciousness.

Understanding the role of gamma waves can enrich your approaches to meditation, guided imagery, and other forms of neurological programming that aim to elevate mental states. Techniques promoting relaxation and mental coherence, such as deep breathing, focused attention, or chanting, can increase gamma wave activity, improving mental agility and psychological well-being.

Gamma waves illustrate the profound connection between advanced brain functions and states of higher consciousness and spirituality, bridging the gap between the scientific and the metaphysical in intriguing ways. The basic tenet of gamma waves is that once reached, there is no longer an ego/personality or a separate identity. This is called the Super Conscious Mind or Universal Consciousness, where perfection is present. Thus, the body is aligned and healed to perfection in this state.

Using Brain Waves

Brainwaves' true potential lies in utilizing them to our advantage. It is fascinating how our brain can become more adept at accessing and using different brainwave states. Techniques like meditation, mindfulness exercises, and self-hypnosis can help us train our brains in this regard. By practicing relaxation techniques and quieting the active thoughts in one's mind, one can reduce stress and improve sleep.

Brainwaves offer insights into the wide range of mental activity and consciousness that we go through in our daily lives. Discovering a whole new realm of possibilities for personal development, enhanced well-being, and a stronger connection to ourselves and the world can be achieved by gaining a deeper understanding of these states and learning how to navigate them. Through consistent practice, we can develop the ability to synchronize our brainwaves and cultivate a life filled with clarity, creativity, inner calm, and healing the body. It's like mastering a complex symphony.

"...a total, deep relaxation level is the most important precondition for curing any disorder. The underlying concept is that the body knows how to maintain balance unless thrown off by disease: if one wants to restore the body's healing ability, everything should be done to bring it back into balance."

– Deepak Chopra, Md, Quantum Healing

Chapter 5:
The Body-Mind Connection

"What the mind knows is also known by the body and DNA. Your experiences resonate on all three levels: mind, body, and DNA. You cannot be happy or sad, sick or well, awake or asleep, without sending a message everywhere in the body."

- Depok Chopra

The 'Second Brain' – the Gut

One of the first things I ask a client is where in the body they experience emotion, fear, anxiety, and all other presenting issues. The body gives me clues about the initial sensitizing event that occurred in their life. This enables me to establish a strategy leading to the release and change of the conflict, resulting in greater harmony in their life.

People are a complicated mix of mind and body; holistic healing understands the complex connection between the two. From this vantage point, it is accepted that the 'mind,' also known as the 'instinctive mind,' oversees and directs our bodies' vital functions. The seat of this instinctive mind is in the Solar Plexus, also sometimes called the 'Abdominal Brain' or the 'Gut Brain.'

The gut-brain connection refers to the bidirectional communication network between the gastrointestinal tract and the central nervous system, called the "gut-brain axis." This connection influences our emotions, thoughts, and overall health. The gut and brain constantly communicate through a complex network of nerves, hormones, and biochemical signals.

Instinct, a primal survival mechanism ingrained in various organisms, primarily serves as a warning signal against danger. It is also important to remember that the subconscious considers everything a threat and will respond to the degree the threat presents, as recorded by the body's nervous system.

"Everything operates on threads and dominos; this is your solar plexus."

– Caroline Myss, Medical Intuitive

The Solar Plexus is inactive in everyday situations. In contrast, it 'wakes up' and becomes active when a significant threat or an urgent need exists. It fights to overcome obstacles and keep the person safe. Stimulating this process can be beneficial. However, it would be best to focus on the present moment.

There are three main ideas at play here:

1. The instinctive mind controls the body's functions and organs.

2. The instinctive mind is in the Solar Plexus or the Abdominal Brain.

3. The instinctive mind can be reached and contacted when the Solar Plexus is stimulated and brought to conscious awareness.

This knowledge could be used to achieve the goal of health control. Poor habits and routines stress organs. The Solar Plexus can work to repair any dysfunctional organ. As the Solar Plexus's instinctive mind works to repair damage, it needs help from the 'thinking mind" to correct unhealthy choices.

"Two general phases, i.e., (1) the phase of Inner States; and (2) the phase of Outer Forms. These two phases, however, are not separate or opposed to each other but are complementary aspects of the same thing. There is always an action and reaction between the Inner State and the Outer Form— between the Inner Feeling and the Outer Expression. If we know the particular Inner State, we may infer the appropriate Outer Form; and if we know the Outer Form, we may infer the Inner State."

- Atkinson, William Walker – How to read human nature

When a person is ready and willing to work with the Solar Plexus to improve their health and biological functioning, the Solar Plexus reacts willingly and even joyfully to their efforts. On the other hand, it is crucial to focus clearly and productively on the organ that isn't working right and its problems. Simply put, the gut, called the Solar Plexus, is a powerful tool for improving health and well-being. Learning how this second brain works and how to connect with it can help our physical well-being, mental health, and wellness.

The Vagus Nerve and the Subconscious Connection

We have a beautiful nerve deep inside our bodies that controls the processes that are most important to us all the time. The vagus nerve goes from the brainstem to the chest and abdomen. It is a long nerve that winds around in different directions. This remarkable nerve is essential to the autonomic nervous system, which controls many of the body's natural functions.

When we look at the vagus nerve, we see that it comprises two nerves, one on each side of the body. It starts its trip in the brainstem, goes through the neck, and finally comes out of the abdominal cavity, the chest, and the abdomen. The vagus nerve is a primary communication pathway between the gut and the brain. Activation of the vagus nerve can influence mood, stress levels, and even inflammation.

It is also in charge of sending sensory information from many organs back to the brain. This gives the brain vital information about the health of our heart, lungs, digestive, and other systems. This nerve is critical for physical health and helps us understand our feelings.

The gut produces many of the same neurotransmitters as the brain, such as serotonin, dopamine, and gamma-aminobutyric acid (GABA). About 90% of the body's serotonin is produced in the gut. Serotonin is associated with happiness, focus, and calmness. Dopamine is associated with rewards and motivation. These neurotransmitters regulate mood, anxiety, and emotional well-being. The gut microbiota, the community of bacteria, fungi, and other microorganisms living in the intestines, is a crucial player in the gut-brain axis.

The microbiota influences brain function and behavior by producing neurotransmitter precursors and modulating inflammation. An imbalance in gut bacteria has been linked to various mental health conditions, such as anxiety, depression, and even cognitive decline. Psychological stress can alter gut function, leading to symptoms like indigestion, bloating, and changes in bowel habits.

Conversely, gut health can affect psychological states. For instance, inflammation in the gut can contribute to symptoms of depression. Diet plays a crucial role in maintaining gut health and, consequently, brain health.

Understanding the gut-brain axis opens new avenues for treating psychological and physiological disorders. Practices such as dietary changes, stress reduction techniques, probiotics, and vagus nerve stimulation can positively impact gut and brain health.

The gut-brain axis represents a holistic system where physical and mental health are deeply intertwined. Therefore, a comprehensive approach that addresses gut and brain function can be more effective in achieving overall well-being.

The vagus nerve's influence extends to nearly every major organ and system in the body. Its health and function are critical in maintaining physical, mental, and emotional well-being. Understanding and supporting vagal function through lifestyle practices, therapies, and mind-body techniques can improve health outcomes and greater resilience against stress and disease.

The Solar Plexus and The Subconscious Mind

The solar plexus, the *third chakra* in energy healing systems, is significantly connected to the subconscious mind. It acts as an energetic and physical center that influences our emotions, intuition, and sense of personal power. This connection manifests through its influence on gut feelings, instincts, and emotions that arise seemingly out of nowhere. The solar plexus is also considered the seat of identity and ego, where feelings of self-worth and confidence are nurtured.

The solar plexus is the center of willpower and autonomy, influencing how we assert ourselves and manage emotions like fear, anger, and joy. It also transmits subconscious signals to the brain, often perceived as "gut instincts" or "gut feelings." The subconscious mind frequently communicates through sensations in the solar plexus region, usually felt as a sense of unease, excitement, or intuition. This is where the phrase "trust your gut" comes from.

The solar plexus is highly responsive to emotional stimuli and stress. When under stress, people often feel a tightness or discomfort in the stomach area. This response is the body's way of processing subconscious emotional information, sometimes linked to unresolved issues, traumas, or suppressed feelings—the solar plexus stores emotional memories, particularly those related to personal identity and power dynamics. Traumatic experiences or unresolved emotions can block the solar plexus, affecting both conscious thought and subconscious reactions. The solar plexus is the center of manifestation in the body, where intention and willpower are transformed into action. When the solar plexus is balanced and healthy, it facilitates clear communication between the conscious desires and the subconscious mind, helping to manifest goals and dreams with confidence.

Strengthen the Vagus Nerve, Solar Plexus, and Subconscious Connection

The solar plexus is more than just an energy center—it's a powerful hub that bridges the conscious mind and subconscious processes. By nurturing the health and balance of the solar plexus, one can enhance personal empowerment, intuition, and subconscious clarity. Stimulating the vagus nerve can have many benefits, including reducing stress, improving mood, and promoting better digestion. It's often activated through practices that help the body achieve a state of relaxation and restoration. Here are several methods to effectively stimulate the powerhouse of our life:

- Diaphragmatic Breathing: Inhale deeply through the nose, expanding your abdomen, and exhale slowly through the mouth. Aim for 4-6 breaths per minute. Deep, slow breathing reduces heart rate and promotes vagal tone, signaling the body to relax.

- Visualizing a calm, peaceful place can also reduce stress, like being in the ocean listening to waves.

- Humming, Chanting, Singing: Chanting or listening to sounds at 528 Hz (associated with the solar plexus) can help balance and activate this energy center. Listening to classical music, where sounds are vibrations, can trigger healing.

- Physical Exercise: Gentle movement practices like yoga and Tai Chi promote relaxation and enhance vagal tone. Poses emphasizing slow breathing and relaxation, such as forward bends or legs-up-the-wall poses, are particularly effective. Moderate physical activity, such as walking, swimming, or cycling, enhances vagus nerve function and parasympathetic activity. Avoid intense, high-impact exercise when working to calm the solar plexus.

- Probiotics and Diet: A balanced diet rich in fiber, omega-3s, and antioxidants can support gut health, indirectly benefiting vagal tone. Diet plays a crucial role in maintaining gut health and, consequently, brain health. Fermented foods, dietary fibers, and probiotics are particularly beneficial for supporting a healthy gut-brain connection.

- Mindfulness or meditation mainly focuses on breath or bodily sensations and stimulates the vagus nerve. Practices like loving-kindness meditation can also promote feelings of compassion and connection.

- Social Connections and Positive Emotions: Social interactions and emotions like laughter stimulate the vagus nerve. Building strong social connections and expressing gratitude or joy enhances the vagal tone and reduces stress.

- Practices such as hypnosis, guided visualization, and meditation can help reprogram subconscious patterns by focusing on the solar plexus area. Visualizing bright yellow light (the color associated with the solar plexus chakra) or using affirmations can support subconscious reprogramming related to self-worth, courage, and personal empowerment.

*"When the individual, however, deliberately turns his conscious attention to the matter and uses his will in connection with the process, then the Cerebrum, or **"thinking brain"** exerts a tremendously increased power and influence over the Solar Plexus, or **"feeling brain."** It can dominate the latter to a great extent, and the latter may be easily trained to accept its "suggestions," its demands, and its commands."*

– William Walker Atkinson

The Changeable Brain

The human brain has an incredible ability to change and adapt, known as neuroplasticity. Because of this one-of-a-kind trait, the brain can rearrange itself and create new neural pathways, allowing us to learn new skills, remember things, and overcome traumas.

Our brains change constantly throughout our lives to accommodate new knowledge and experiences. As we learn new things, more connections are made between neurons in our brains, which form a neural pathway. This pathway will only strengthen through repeated practice and reinforcement of this newly learned skill or information.

Still, our brains can become very good at keeping us safe, making us hyperaware and tense even when there isn't a real threat. In cases like these, exercises that emphasize neuroplasticity can help reduce anxiety. By learning new behaviors and thoughts, we can *rewire* our brains to react differently to things that make us anxious. This enables us to weaken and create new neural pathways.

Self-Directed Neuroplasticity

Self-directed neuroplasticity means people can consciously rewire their brains to break bad habits and create new ones. It is based on the idea that a person's brain is malleable and can change throughout their lives.

Neurons transmit information between each other through chemical and electrical signals via synapses, thereby forming neural networks, which are a series of interconnected neurons. This is meant by "the wiring of the brain" and "neurons that fire together, wire together."

The human brain is wired to adapt to the environment's requirements for survival. Today and in the future, it will not be as important to internalize information as to be elastically able to take in multiple sources of information, synthesize them, and make rapid decisions.

Our brains are always changing in response to new knowledge and experiences. This creates neural pathways that help us learn new skills, remember things, and respond to our surroundings. However, these neural pathways can sometimes become set, leading to bad habits that are hard to change.

Self-directed neuroplasticity can help address this problem. By practicing new behaviors and thoughts on purpose, people can rewire their brains to react differently to things that set off bad habits. They can use this to create new neural pathways and weaken old ones.

This idea is used all the time to help someone change a habit like smoking cigarettes. They can do this by developing new behaviors and thoughts that are incompatible with smoking. This means responding differently to emotions that trigger and urge them to smoke. Taking new actions to address stressors and emotions triggers the brain to recognize new behavior patterns and begin rewiring.

You can use this method to encourage the behavior. Mindfulness and meditation are just a few ways to help people create new neural pathways that make it easier to change mindsets, even when stressed or distracted.

Mindfulness empowers people to control their brain function and make changes that matter to them. If people break bad habits and create good ones, their mental and physical health will improve, they will be more productive, and their overall well-being will improve.

Self-directed neuroplasticity helps people become stronger and more flexible when things go wrong, or their lives change. By actively rewiring our brains, we can develop new skills, perspectives, and ways of thinking that help us deal with the challenges of modern life more comfortably and confidently. This can be paramount to healing the body via the mind link.

"A major study of four hundred spontaneous remissions of cancer found that all the patients had only one thing in common: the person had changed his attitudes before the remission occurred, finding some way to become hopeful, courageous, and positive."

– Quantum Healing, Dr. Depok Copra

The Living Brain

Instead of being a passive vessel that we fill with information, the brain is a living organ that changes and grows when it gets the right food and exercise. The brain changes physically because of the decisions we make and the actions we take daily.

The environment where we grow up significantly affects how our brains develop. Philosopher Jim Rohn said, *"You are the average of the five people you spend the most time with."* This is because our brains constantly change in response to the information and behaviors of those around us.

As observers, we are separate from our brains and can choose what thoughts to accept or reject. The most important thing to remember about learning how to respond to life is that the brain is hardwired to adapt to meet the needs of our surroundings and stay alive. Thanks to progress in genetic technology, we may one day be able to teach brain cells to make new types of chemical signals and receptors. This may allow us to create personalities with specific traits.

Neurogenesis is the process by which the brain changes over a person's life. It is an integral part of neuroplasticity. New connections are made between brain cells, changing and improving cognition. If someone's thinking mind is changed in a way that brings back balance and unity, these new pathways can also heal your body.

"We casually assume that a person who survives cancer or can cure himself of a fatal disease operates with the same mental machinery as anyone else, but this is not true: mental processes can be deep or shallow. To go deep means to contact the hidden blueprint of intelligence and change it – only then can visualization of fighting cancer be strong enough to defeat the disease."

– Depok Chopra, Quantum Healing

I have observed that this level of healing demands a high degree of meditation or Hypnosis to reach the gamma and other brain waves that make this possible. I have helped clients reach this level through hypnosis, which allows them to connect to a personal higher source that provides important information.

Neurons to the rescue. A type of cell that receives and sends messages from the body to the brain and back to the body. The messages are sent by a weak electrical current called a nerve cell. Neurons fire when a person visualizes or sees someone else take an appealing action. If there is value in the action, it is then wired into their brain.

The Hebbian Theory

In 1949, a Canadian scientist named Donald Hebb developed an idea that would change how we think about the brain's ability to learn and change. In Hebb's postulate, synaptic connections between neurons (brain cells) could be made stronger by activating them often and for a long time. This is one of the most essential ideas in neuroscience, and it forms the basis of a way of learning called Hebbian learning. Donald Hebb said it best: *"Neurons that fire together, wire together."* This simple idea can have enormous and far-reaching effects.

Hebbian learning is all about associative learning. When many cells are activated simultaneously, the synapse strength between those cells gets much stronger. This is why the connection between two neurons gets more robust when they are both stimulated at the same time. This connection is known as "mirror neurons." Neurons that wire together create many different types of learning and memory, including picking up new skills.

Brain cells known as 'mirror neurons' allow information and behavior to be transmitted from one person to another via the 'neural WiFi' phenomenon. Mirror neurons are one of the most critical parts of Hebbian learning. They help us understand the actions of others by mirroring those actions in our neural circuits. These neurons play a role in learning through imitation. When we observe others' actions, our mirror neurons can activate as though we are taking the same action, which helps us understand and mimic new behaviors.

Mirror neurons may contribute to our ability to empathize with others, allowing us to simulate another person's emotions, pain, or intentions within our brain. They may also be involved in language acquisition and development, as they could enable individuals to understand and replicate the gestures and sounds they observe in others.

Additionally, Hebbian learning helps make synaptic connections between simultaneously activated cells. When an animal watches another animal take a particular action, mirror neurons fire in the observer's brain, forming a new neural link for a more preferred action.

Along with the power of Hebbian learning and mirror neurons, visualization methods, like those used in Hypnosis and Neuro-Linguistic Programming (NLP). These interventions work by having the person imagine a happy experience to change a bad experience. When someone re-experiences the emotions and feelings they want and imagine themselves in the new experience, their physical senses are heightened, and their brain creates new neural connections.

"The world we have created is a process of our thinking. It cannot be changed without changing our thinking."

– Albert Einstein

Combining these two experiences allows the mind to accept the most positive experience and rewires itself. Dismissing the old experience and replacing it with a new, more positive experience is a great way to change bad habits or emotional responses that no longer fit our preferred actions.

"I visualize things in my mind before I have to do them. It's like having a mental workshop."

– Jack Youngblood

In therapeutic role-play or guided journeys, asking a client to imagine themselves in another person's position (e.g., seeing the situation from the perspective of a loved one or their higher self) can stimulate mirror neurons, leading to significant shifts in perception and enhanced empathy.

"Your beliefs become your thoughts, thoughts become your words, your words become your actions, your actions become your habits, your habits become your values, and your values become your destiny."

– Mahatma Gandhi

Bad habits are the response to *negative* emotions that act as the cue connecting the response and the reward in the brain. Once the subconscious recognizes the change in the body that produces consistent action, these become the default circuits. On the other hand, focused attention and practice can change the brain's reward system to make bad habits less appealing and replace them with better behavior patterns.

"Anytime you're gonna grow, you're gonna lose something. You're losing what you're hanging onto to keep safe. You're losing habits that you're comfortable with, you're losing familiarity."

- James Hillman

To change habits, you must repeatedly adopt new actions. When we consistently take a different action, the subconscious recognizes this new response to an old message via the body. Our nerve cells then literally create new connections between nerve centers. Eventually, this turns into a preferred choice.

Remember that changing habits and learning new skills generally require between twenty and thirty days for the subconscious to support the change. I have experienced this, having helped hundreds of clients stop smoking. The subconscious mind never forgets a habit. The subconscious responds to new behaviors unless the old behavior is slightly reintroduced.

"There is no such thing as good habits and bad habits. Habit means living life without awareness."

– Sadhguru

Tools for Change

Many of our beliefs and assumptions are unconscious. They were absorbed without much thought, learned when we were young, and picked up without our awareness. Since our unconscious beliefs have stayed the same, we make the same mistakes.

We need to connect with our subconscious mind to change our habits. This will make it possible for us to make changes. Our feelings, emotions, and regular behavior patterns come from our subconscious mind, which is always in touch with our resources and abilities. If we want to change our habits, we need to re-program our subconscious mind with new beliefs and ideas that are empowering, hopeful, and positive.

Affirmations can help us change our subconscious mind to be more upbeat. An affirmation is when we repeatedly say good things to ourselves to help us believe these thoughts and beliefs are true. Daily mantras can help you change how you think and feel over time. You may then change your habits and behaviors.

"The mind is a primary determinant of the body's health, and simple interventions to change the way we think can dramatically improve our well-being."

– Dr. Ellen Langer, Social Psychologist

Our minds shape what we experience. Our most valuable assets as human beings are the ability to use 'imagination' and 'visualization.' Through imagination, we can generate new ideas and thoughts, and through visualization, we can bring those ideas to life.

Our imaginations come from our conscious minds, so we can think of anything, even if it's false. Our thoughts and feelings can make our bodies react because our subconscious mind can't tell the difference between what is real and what is imagined. For example, when we think about a scary situation, our bodies may behave as if it were happening. This is what sets off the fight-or-flight response.

However, we can all use visualization to create the life we choose. If we focus on the good things that will happen and picture ourselves reaching our goals, we can use the power of our subconscious mind to make these images come true. Negative visualizations can also create a world we don't want to be a part of, so it's important to be aware of our thoughts and feelings.

"Visualize the thing you want, see, feel, and believe in. Make your mental blueprint and begin to build. "

– Robert Collier

Our subconscious controls our long-term memories, habits, emotions, and behaviors. It is a digital library of all our memories, connecting all our events to the ones that came before them. Our subconscious mind constantly scans our surroundings for possible real or imagined threats to ensure our safety and security.

In addition, our mental pictures of what we want will set off chemical processes in our minds and bodies. This is the job of the subconscious mind. When we picture reaching our goals, our subconscious mind creates new neural pathways and sends signals to our body's organs. This turns on the proprioceptive field (sometimes called the "auric field"), the external electrical field surrounding our physical bodies. This is the concept of attraction, repulsion, adhesion, and cohesion in our lives.

Luther Burbank cited, *"Heredity is a powerful factor because it gives the will to work with raw material."* If there is no substance, not even willpower can make something happen. The subconscious mind is the one that makes things happen, and it knows how to help us lead and direct our lives. It creates chemical reactions to answer our ideas about what we want. If we use the power of our subconscious mind, we can become the creative principle. Which means we must be responsible for everything in our world.

Our imagination and visualization skills are powerful tools that can change how we see the world. Being aware of our thoughts and feelings and using visualization as a tool for change can help us tap into the power of our subconscious mind to create the life we choose. By understanding how powerful we and our subconscious mind are, we can control our lives and create the reality we choose to experience.

"Whatever the mind of man can conceive and believe, it can achieve."

– Napolean Hill

Chapter 6:
Liberating The Mind

"We casually assume that a person who survives cancer or can cure himself of a fatal disease operates with the same mental machinery as anyone else, but this is not true: mental processes can be deep or shallow. To go deep means to contact the hidden blueprint of intelligence and change it – only then can visualization of fighting cancer be strong enough to defeat the disease."

– Dr. Ellen Langer, Social Psychologist at Harvard

Most of us have been stuck in a never-ending loop of negative emotions and thoughts. Imagine a world where these things do not limit you, and you can fully embrace the present moment with absolute clarity and presence. Let us begin by exploring a broader definition of healing that acknowledges the powerful influence of the mind on our well-being. We will dive into the inner workings of fear and how it can stem from our own limiting beliefs. You will be able to respond consciously instead of reacting impulsively by learning to differentiate between fleeting feelings and complex emotions. One of the main objectives behind this technique is to help you shift negative thought patterns and develop the ability to objectively monitor your feelings and emotions. Finally, no healing can be had without Soul, Mind, and Body alignment.

Fear and the Mind

Fear interferes with our thoughts and decision-making by making us uncertain. Fear can profoundly impact the mind and body, influencing behavior, emotions, and physical health. When we get scared, we usually fixate on a situation's potential downsides instead of considering its positive opportunities. This can result in a never-ending loop of anxiety, stress, and depression, which can hold us back and make it difficult to act.

Fear often leads to feelings of anxiety, making individuals feel overwhelmed or tense. Intense fear can cause panic attacks, which can lead to a loss of control over emotions and physical responses. Fear triggers the fight-or-flight response, either hyperactivity (fighting or fleeing) or emotional paralysis (freezing).

Fear releases adrenaline and cortisol, which prepare the body to respond to a threat. Long-term exposure to these hormones can negatively impact health, leading to conditions such as hypertension, cardiovascular disease, or weakened immunity. The body's autonomic nervous system speeds up heart rate and breathing, preparing for quick action. Muscles often tighten, leading to chronic tension, headaches, or back pain. These are common physical manifestations when the body senses danger.

Fear can cloud judgment, making reasoning or sound decisions difficult. It can also lead to constantly scanning the environment for threats, making it difficult to relax. Chronic fear may impair the brain's ability to form new memories or recall previous experiences.

Fear often leads to avoiding situations, people, or challenges that trigger anxiety. This can limit personal growth or create phobias. Sometimes, fear triggers aggressive responses as a defense mechanism. Fear can lead people to withdraw from social situations or retreat into isolation.

"If you made a list of 101 Fears, they would represent 101 conditions, situations, and things which have no existence .... except in your mind.

– John Randolph Price, Angels Among Us, Angel of Love & Freedom

Fear arises when we live in our minds instead of in the moment without negative emotion—except what life offers. Fear often seems to result from our thoughts and perceptions rather than something objectively real.

From a metaphysical or spiritual perspective, fear can block energy flow within the body, leading to stagnation or imbalance in the body's energy centers (chakras). Fear may lead to disconnection from one's spiritual path or higher purpose, creating a sense of isolation or disempowerment.

Over time, prolonged exposure to fear can diminish one's overall well-being, limiting the capacity to experience joy, peace, or fulfillment. In many spiritual and psychological healing traditions, addressing fear is critical to unlocking deeper self-awareness and growth.

"Look at your fears; ...anything you could be afraid of is nothing but an "effect"…. including people, places, and things."

– Dr. David Hawkins

Past experiences influence fear, shaping our beliefs and expectations about the world. Our emotions are always connected to our desires and nothing else. Our fears are often linked to what we want and expect and can be set off by things threatening those desires. For instance, if we have been through tough times or suffered a loss, we might feel scared of going through something similar again. Even when we were forty, the event happened as a teenager or earlier.

"One is not ruled by the mind at all. The mind reveals endless options disguised as memories, fantasies, fears, concepts, etc. To get free of domination by the mind, it is only necessary to realize that its parade of subjects is merely an arbitrary cafeteria of selections winding their way across the screen of the mind."

– Dr. David Hawkins

Incorrect ideas and misunderstandings can also increase fear. Our understanding of reality is sometimes limited and personal, and our preconceptions and preferences can shape it. When we cling to incorrect beliefs or misunderstandings, we can feel scared and unsure about things that are not true.

The ego is a defense mechanism designed to ensure survival at all costs. It is proficient at denying its failings and inferiorities, suppressing these rejected aspects into the unconscious mind and thus denying them expression. Once this is done, it must still find expression through projection, usually onto someone else. When things become rigid and inflexible, adapting to changing circumstances can make it challenging.

"False Self (ego)...little more than a collection of habits coalesces to form a rigid identity, with no creativity, intuition, ability to experiment, and little connection to the body and its feelings. It focuses on outside approval, appearances, money, security, and social standing. It seeks established methods and protocols for guidance, becoming extremely fearful in novel situations – hence its relentless efforts to keep everything under control and move according to well-worn patterns."

- Linda Kohanov, Ways of the Horse

But do you know what? You can conquer fear and start living a good life of fulfillment and empowerment while living in the NOW! This moment. NOW is all there is. It is a tall task, but this moment is the only time a feeling or decision can be made. If we tap into this incredible power and potential, we can conquer fear and live authentic, fulfilling lives for and with each other.

"... As we are liberated from our fear, our presence automatically liberates others."

– Mariann Williamson

Fear is a normal part of being human, but we can rise above it and move forward. By better grasping what makes us fearful and facing our made-up stories of "what may be, might be, could be, or should be." These are all lies made up in the mind. We are co-creators, and we were never born to "should." Fear is often a result of how we see things and our choices. We can choose to defeat fear with courage. It only takes twenty seconds to be a hero. Face the fear and become free.

Hypnosis and NLP Benefits

Rewiring our brains through hypnosis is an effective way to tackle fear. By identifying and reworking the neural pathways associated with fear, we can create new patterns of thought and behavior, leading to a more empowering and positive mindset. It is all about changing how we see things.

Hypnosis is a state of deep relaxation and focused attention. In this state, the conscious mind becomes quiet, allowing the subconscious mind to become more accessible. Since all fears are subconscious and memory, hypnosis can reprogram automatic fear responses or irrational thought patterns.

Neurolinguistic Programming (NLP) works against fear using our most powerful tool, visualization. Visualizing an image of courage while seeing oneself involved in an event of fear can give us the strength to face fear from a different perspective and belief. I had a 7-year-old client fearful of spiders. Ever since seeing one in the bathtub, he wouldn't take a bath or shower. I had him tell me his favorite hero, which turned out to be Mighty Mouse. I inquired if Might Mouse was afraid of spiders. He assured me he was not and that Mighty Mouse was his friend and would protect him from spiders. Seeing himself taking a shower with Mighty Mouse's protection, his mother informed me he could shower the next day and after that.

Hypnosis and NLP use guided imagery, leading a person through a peaceful or empowering visualization. For example, someone who fears flying might be guided to imagine themselves safely and calmly boarding a plane and enjoying the flight without anxiety. This practice allows the subconscious mind to experience the feared situation calmly and in control, helping desensitize the person to the fear.

While under hypnosis, the individual can receive positive suggestions that help reframe their fearful responses. For example, if someone is afraid of public speaking, the hypnotherapist might offer suggestions connected to a time when one was supremely confident. Then, the person could use that confidence in speaking and replace the fear with a peaceful presentation. Suggestions interrupt the fear cycle and replace it with more rational or positive responses when the person encounters the feared situation.

Through Hypnosis and NLP, we can discover and eliminate the root causes of fear, reprogram our responses, and introduce calming suggestions. Whether used alone or alongside other therapeutic techniques, hypnosis is a powerful tool for transforming fear into confidence and empowerment.

Building self-confidence and inner strength is crucial for overcoming fear. A hypnotherapist may provide affirmations and positive suggestions to strengthen the person's belief in their ability to manage the feared situation with guidance where there was self-confidence in another situation yet connecting it to a fearful situation.

One technique involves creating an anchor of a positive experience and connecting it to the fearful experience. Once the two experiences are connected, the subconscious will always choose the response that makes one feel better over the negative response. For example, the hypnotherapist might help the person associate a calm feeling with a simple action like pressing their thumb and forefinger together. When fear arises, they can use this anchor to trigger the relaxed state they experienced during hypnosis.

In hypnosis, the person may be guided to view their fear from a distance or in a detached way. By mentally dissociating from the fear, they can observe it without emotional reaction, weakening its control over their response. This allows the person to experience fear or anxiety as an observer, reducing the intensity and bringing about a more normal preferred response. Known as a desensitization technique, the person is gradually exposed to their fear in small, manageable steps while remaining relaxed, ultimately eliminating the fearful event and response.

Difference between Feelings and Emotions

"We live in feelings, not in figures on a sundial. We should count time in heartbeats."

– Aristotle

There are two ways to evaluate truth in our lives: feelings and emotions. Human beings are naturally emotive creatures. We often talk about how we are feeling. Over lifetimes, we experience millions of different sensations. We will be touched by feelings and emotions every day. Frequently, these two terms are used interchangeably, but there are differences between feelings and emotions that, if known, can help us better understand what is going on inside.

The definition of feeling refers to something experienced by outside stimuli reacting with one of your senses, sensibilities, attitude, or perception. Feelings are experienced for short periods, moment-to-moment. If you touch a stove, it feels hot, and you quickly remove your hand. If someone jumps out at you from around a corner, you will feel startled, but that will soon pass. Feelings of excitement will subside after the event is done.

"When you choose a combination of thoughts and feelings, you offer a signal that has never been offered before. And so, the Universe must uniquely yield to you, which causes you to offer a vibration that maybe

someone somewhere else is matching. If they are, they will certainly come into your experience for the matching time." That is the way you affect the world. You affect the world by achieving the vibration that brings the signals to you. You create a nucleus that the Universe has to respond to. That is how you are the creator.

– Abraham Hicks

Likewise, an emotion is technically a state of consciousness in which various internal sensations are experienced. Because of this, the most significant difference between feelings and emotions is that an external motivating factor must trigger feelings, whereas emotions can be completely internalized. Emotions are produced by a thought, memory, or external motivator and often change our physical state.

"Our conscious and unconscious thoughts, emotions, and intents create reality. When they are aligned, we become the reality that we prefer, as long as we are following our excitement, which represents the natural flow of the universe."

– Lyssa Royal Holt, Mystic; Galactic Heritage Tarot

Emotions serve specific purposes; they help us set priorities and shape our physical and mental experiences. Your emotions are always about your relationship with your desire and nothing else. Emotions are long-term states. If you are in love and joyful, that emotion will usually last years. Sorrow, too, takes a long time to go away. Because emotions are internal, you must change your mindset to change your emotions, which sometimes takes time. Understanding the difference between feelings and emotions can help us respond to situations with greater self-awareness. We decide how to react when we respond to life with negative emotions. We must understand that there is a belief that supports emotion, which may or may not be accurate.

103

"Emotions are always true – they always tell the truth about how you are feeling."

– Karla McLaren, Language of Emotions

The obstacle between you and your well-being is letting external influences guide your thoughts and emotions instead of your deepest, most authentic part of yourself—your core identity beyond external roles, expectations, or influences. It includes our unique values, desires, intuitive wisdom, and inner voice, reflecting who we are at a soul or essence level. Unlike the outer self, shaped by societal conditioning, the inner self is the source of inner knowing, self-awareness, and guidance that aligns with our true nature.

For instance, when we experience anger, we can take a deep breath and pause before responding. When we know what we are feeling, we can take the time to dig deeper and figure out why we are feeling that way. Knowing the distinction between feelings and emotions can assist us in responding to situations with greater awareness and making deliberate decisions.

"As spiritual awareness advances, the flow of spiritual energy increases and enables transcending prior, seemingly insurmountable obstacles. As the attractions of the world and emotions decrease, there is a progressive attraction to qualities such as beauty, lovability, and peace, rather than "things" or seeming gains."

– Dr. David Hawkins

When we take the time to tune in to our feelings and emotions, we can gain a deeper understanding of our authentic selves by evaluating our thoughts and beliefs based on an experience.

The Liberation of Emotions

"Everything we shut our eyes to, everything we run away from, everything we deny, denigrate, or despise, serves to defeat us in the end. What seems nasty, painful, evil can become a source of beauty, joy, and strength if faced with an open mind."

-Henry Miller

Emotions play a significant role in expanding our awareness and nurturing our emotional and spiritual growth. Feelings drive progress, add excitement and vibrancy to our lives, infuse our endeavors and actions with energy, inspire innovation, and deepen our sense of purpose and spirituality. On the other hand, our negative emotions can influence how we respond to life. It is essential to assess your beliefs vs. what is true.

Examining fear can make us anxious and cause us to avoid certain situations. To manage our emotions, we must be mindful of any tendencies to deny or control them as we process them. Emotional digestion is about taking our negative emotions and turning them into positive options to act upon. This allows us to be more natural in our response to life. Emotional work involves balancing the body, mind, emotions, and spirituality. Addressing the subconscious dominance of emotions is essential, as it can be the root cause of many issues.

"It is possible that there might not be a more fundamental psychological skill than the control of impulses. Impulse control is the basis of all emotional self-control because every emotion is known to cause an impulse of action."

– Sigmund Freud

Early programming may often lead to controlling our emotions as a child, which does not allow us to express ourselves fully. This led to suppression. And you know what happens when things get suppressed - they always find a way to resurface. This causes a buildup of energy that comes out in numerous ways, redefining who we naturally are, and that causes multiple unnatural characteristics. Such as helplessness, bitterness, jealousy, depression, and distrust, to name a few negative responses to life.

Go back, through memory, to when things went wrong. This is where you can heal. We find healing by reconnecting within that situation and seeing our innate, instinctive response situation again. For instance, we shed tears when feeling down, stomp our feet, whack a pillow with a carpet beater, shout when we are mad, seek security when we are frightened, and burst into laughter when we are joyful.

"When emotions are pent up, you lose the ability to express yourself naturally and spontaneously. You can only be spontaneous if you fully accept yourself. Letting go of control over yourself hinders spontaneous expression. You encounter guilt, shame, doubt, and self-hatred, but liberation offers release and allows the inner child to express it. In a safe environment, you return to natural impulses; you can become spontaneous again. Once, you were natural and responded naturally when you were a child."

– Riet Okken, The Liberating Power of Emotions

To sum up, if we want to break free from false beliefs holding us back, we must address our fears, surrender them, and have faith in something more significant. It is essential to align our desires with a higher purpose, handle and process our emotions, acknowledge denial or need for control, and turn negative emotions into opportunities to redefine our thoughts and beliefs to create the reality we choose. If we take ownership of our feelings and emotions, we can find healing and reconnect with our authentic, instinctive selves. By doing that, we can break free from our fears, discover our true desires, and find emotional liberation.

"There can be no transforming of darkness into light and of apathy (state of suppressed emotions; indifference;) into movement without EMOTION!"

– C.G. Jung

Exercise for Thinking and Feeling

Arousal Exercise:

1. Hyperventilate by breathing heavily for a few seconds. STOP! Close your eyes. Notice what your body feels like. Make a mental note of all the sensations.

2. Run in place for a minute or two.

3. Think and focus on something very upsetting and put it in the palm of one hand. Now, scan the body and notice the heaviness of the thought. Where is the body more tense or heavier? Now dump it out.

4. Think about something exciting. Scan the body, notice the lightness in your hand, and observe how the body responds and feels. Put your hands together and cover your heart with your palms. Notice how you feel.

Reflection:

Notice what is happening inside your body. Take a moment to focus on the present moment and identify the physical sensations you are experiencing. Observe these sensations objectively, without judgment. Ask yourself: *"What am I feeling in my body right now?"* *"Where do I feel it?"* *"What does it feel like?"*

The exercise aims to recognize how our thoughts and feelings affect our bodies. A belief and emotion that has a history in your life easily leads to disharmony in the body. The body is the final arbiter of truth in thinking.

Relaxation Exercise:

Close your eyes and exhale deeply. Let your shoulders drop. Rotate your head gently and loosely until you find a comfortable, balanced position for your head, neck, and shoulders. Let your jaw relax and hang loose. Relax your lips, tongue, and throat. I exhale deeply a few times. Open your eyes.

Reflection:

STOP! Now relax. Notice what your body feels like. Make a mental note of all the sensations. Compare these to the sensations you noticed when you did the arousal exercises. Take a moment to reflect on how your body feels in this relaxed state. Ask yourself: *"What am I feeling in my body right now?"* *"How is it different from when I was aroused?"*

Guided Fantasy to Meditation:

1. Relaxation: comfortable position. Breathe, allow mind & body to relax.

2. Image a beautiful scene. Imagery produces alpha waves.

3. Guided fantasy: visualize positive images or scenarios. This produces theta waves.

4. The silence...produces the experience of meditation and being in the moment.

Reflection:

Validate every insight, every flare of subconscious imagery that arises to consciousness, every moment of internal stillness and peace. Know that when this happens, you are meditating! Afterward, take a moment to reflect on any thoughts or feelings that arose during this meditation. *"What am I thinking/feeling right now?" "Is there a negative thought pattern associated with this feeling?" "Can I reframe this thought more positively or neutrally?"*

This exercise helps to bridge the gap between how we think and feel by:

- Focusing on the present moment and identifying physical sensations in the body

- Observing these sensations objectively, without judgment

- Identifying feelings and thoughts associated with these sensations.

- Potentially reframing negative thoughts associated with these feelings.

- Cultivating a sense of relaxation and inner peace through guided fantasy and meditation.

NLP Technique – Ability to Focus & Heal

You can do this yourself or have someone read it slowly, acknowledging each step with a head nod.

Healing White Light

Take five deep breaths. On the last breath, hold it for two seconds, let it out, and close your eyes.

1. Imagine/visualize or think about a white light running from the top of your head straight down to the bottom of your spine.

2. Confirm (head nod).

3. Now, turn your total attention to your right shoulder.

4. Get a sense of the distance the right shoulder is to the center light.

5. Confirm (head nod).

6. Now, turn your total attention to the left shoulder.

7. Get a sense of the distance the left shoulder is to the center light.

8. Confirm (head nod).

9. Now, focus on both shoulders.

10. Notice...is it the left shoulder or the right shoulder that seems closer or farther away than the other? (you should identify one or the other 98% of the time)

11. Now, focus on both shoulders and see them exactly the same distance apart.

12. Once the adjustment is made...take a deep breath and open your eyes.

13. Did you notice a shift in reality?

This technique bypasses the critical mind, producing an alpha state and measuring focus and compliance. Once the light is imagined, the theta state is achieved.

In this state, a focused mind activates the healing ability of the subconscious mind, and the shoulders become an equal distance apart.

Congratulations, the subconscious healed the body!

The vision of white light down the body produces a centering effect, balance, and harmony. I have often used this, which is my preferred suggestibility and evaluation with new clients. It reinforces the power of the mind while teaching a client the power of focusing on a body part that is causing pain or trouble.

"A focused mind is one of the most powerful energies in the universe."

– Victor Hansen, Chicken Soup for the Soul

Chapter 7:
Changing Programming And Conditioning

"Man's task is to become conscious of the contents that press upward from the unconscious."

– Carl Jung

Our most significant secret is what's in our subconscious mind. Have you ever wondered why you react the way you do in certain situations or hold on to certain beliefs and values? As you have learned, the subconscious mind is the memory of our existence, now and in our past.

When we are born, we assume we are a blank slate. Nothing could be further from the truth. Through many regressions into past lives, I have learned that we come in with a complete plan for how we will experience life—every detail down to the people involved in our life's journey. Edgar Cayce, in one of his writings, noted that we rarely met a new person in a lifetime—one or two at the most. Soul evolution is the primary goal of a lifetime. So, the script for our life must be patterned and programmed.

We are born completely innocent and, therefore, believe everything. The subconscious mind learns our program through imitation, association, and mimicry. Every encounter throughout our life is a sacred part of our journey. Our responsibility is to take the conditioning and programming into our lives to unravel and find our authentic being.

Who is that? The real you are not pushed by what society thinks, what others expect, and the pressures around you. It is the center of you—your true self, in line with what you care about, what excites you, and your goals. People often say that the authentic self is the simplest form of you, not affected by the fronts or parts you may take on to be accepted or liked by people.

Conditioning and Programming in the Subconscious

The subconscious mind is a big, powerful part of the mind that works below what we notice. It stores information, patterns, and rules that shape how we act, think, feel, and live. This is different from the conscious mind, which makes logic and choices on purpose. The subconscious mind takes information and works instantly, affecting our thoughts and actions.

Strong beliefs about ourselves, others, and the world often start young and shape how we see things. The subconscious stores experiences from early life, families, and society's rules around us. It also stores learned behaviors from parents, teachers, and peers, which affect how we act without thinking.

Old patterns from past lives or situations come back as repeated struggles or feelings that help teach or heal us. These behave like "scripts" until we know them and decide to change or let go. All our memories—even ones we are not aware of now—are hidden away, including sound and bad experiences, including trauma; these affect how we behave today, often without knowing why.

Feelings linked to past events go into the subconscious. The subconscious holds emotions like fear and anger; triggers can be people or events, often without our knowledge. The mind reacts fast based on these feelings, changing moods and actions tied to earlier emotional learning. It also controls regular thought habits such as self-doubt, limiting what we can do.

The subconscious handles information quickly, picking up signs missed by the thinking mind. Gut feelings help guide efforts; intuition links to more profound wisdom beyond logic, giving insights into the paths ahead.

Fear programs to protect us, based on earlier happenings where we might have felt in danger, pushed away, or unsafe. These programs can show up as fight-or-flight actions, avoidance, or defensive moves when we are triggered by prior hurt or trauma. The subconscious might also set up shields, like negative beliefs or emotional walls, that stop us from trying new things or changing our lives when it thinks those changes are risky, even if they could benefit us later.

The subconscious acts as a link to deeper spiritual areas and the group unconscious. It can hold universal energies, signs, and shared memories, linking us to a more significant human experience and spiritual knowledge. These universal symbols may emerge in dreams, visions, or coincidences, giving clues about themes and patterns beyond individual lives. It could also store details about our soul's path, aim, and lessons to steer us through feelings or spiritual understandings towards growth and finding balance with our higher self.

In short, the subconscious mind is a big storage area that affects how we act, see things, and feel. It works most of the time automatically without notice until there is a problem. Meditation, hypnosis, shadow work, and other spiritual or healing methods can change the subconscious to align with consciously choosing to be and move past unhelpful old habits.

Basic self-awareness starts young, but understanding deeper patterns often happens later in life thanks to introspection or spiritual growth gained via experiences like therapy or significant life events that reveal deep-rooted habits.

To wrap up, while self-awareness kicks off around age 2, complete conscious understanding—especially concerning subconscious patterns—often develops during the teen years onward with continued personal growth throughout life.

Astrology Insight

In the mid-eighties, I began my studies of Astrology and past life regressions while exploring the readings at the Edgar Cayce Foundation. Edgar Cayce was considered the sleeping prophet and the most profound channel of the twentieth century. His foundation houses over fourteen thousand readings, most for healing and soul journeys. He would suggest what the soul needed to learn to maximize their lifetime. There was also an understanding of success and failures in a person's life. Studies of such profound information were my seed for Soul Fusion with Universal Consciousness.

"Whether or not we believe in survival of consciousness after death, reincarnation, and karma, it has severe implications for our behavior."

– Stanislav Grof

This experience started my passionate study of Astrology, an energy map erected for the moment of birth. It reveals vast information about your soul's journey's past, present, and spiritual path.

A compelling study is the area of the map called the 12th house that defines the subconscious mind's content—often considered one of the most complex and enigmatic areas of the natal chart. This is where the subconscious mind is represented, and this placement reveals incomplete business from the past.

"Who has fully realized that history is not contained in thick books but lives in our very blood."

– Carl Jung

The revelations of this placement and energy are associated with many themes related to the subconscious mind, hidden aspects of life, and spiritual matters. I have witnessed clients gain a profound understanding of their lives and why their life path is the way it is. Conditioning, programs, and past experiences significantly impact how you grow intellectually, behaviorally, and personally. Our values and this placement and energy can all be very healing.

Overall, this is a profoundly introspective area of an individual's map, emphasizing the importance of inner work, spiritual connection, and addressing unresolved issues from the past. It invites individuals to embrace solitude, understand their motivations, and the need to transcend limitations through compassion, healing, and spiritual practice.

Evaluating the 4th house of the Astrological map would complete an understanding. This is where the primary conditioning and programming began in this lifetime. It is the area of family and home. It symbolizes the very roots of our earthly journey—the beginning of life.

This area represents one's physical and internal home, living environment, and the sense of security it provides. It reflects the emotional atmosphere of one's upbringing and family dynamics. This placement speaks to the influence of childhood, including the roots and foundation that shape a person's life.

The fourth house is tied to one's family lineage, heritage, and ancestry. It symbolizes the relationship with parents, particularly the mother or nurturing parent. Traditions, family values, and the influence of ancestors are recognized for their role in shaping a person's identity.

This placement represents a person's inner and outer sanctuary. Emotions, stability, and security are part of the foundations we start with in life. Here, we obtain, among other things, our self-image. It reflects a person's need for privacy and indicates how one retreats, relaxes, and finds comfort in solitude or familiar environments.

Significant influences affect how these themes manifest in a person's life. It forms the foundation of one's emotional well-being and represents the base upon which one builds and maintains one's identity and sense of security throughout life.

In interpretation, this area produces strong opinions from clients, good or bad. Still, I always note that no matter the perspective or opinion, it always shows how the foundation sets up the opportunities for success in a person's life journey.

"For, know that each soul constantly meets itself. No problem may be run away from. Meet it now!"

– Edgar Cayce

Hypnosis Insight

"If you want to know the past, look at the present; if you want to know the future, look at the present."

– Buddha

In my hypnosis work, I gathered many insights into personal conflicts. Age regression is a hypnotist tool that helps clients travel back to an earlier time in their lives, where the early life memories are still causing pain. Insight can be gained about relationships, health issues, spiritual issues, and many others. By revisiting the past, a new perspective can be had from a more mature adult view, no longer seeing events from a child's perspective. By going through the challenging process, we can free ourselves from old memories with new values while releasing the pain and fear deep inside.

The real issue is not that we are conditioned and programmed but whether we choose to heal from them. Then, conditioning and programming become an opportunity to heal. We gain insight into ourselves, get a new perspective, let go of judgment and release the pain and guilt we have held on to from the first conditioning programming stage.

"Healing in the present moment involves resolving the unfinished business of the past, which continues to influence a person in the present moment. Past events' residual mental, emotional, physical, and spiritual energy contaminates the present experience. Resolving the removal of burdensome energies is the goal of any healing approach. Then a person can live more fully in the present and fulfill more completely the details of the life plan that was arranged before the present incarnation."

– William J Baldwin

Healing from Childhood Conditioning

Simply put, it is the difference between the ego/personality and the perfection of being or God-consciousness. Taking responsibility allows us to change perception and perspective, where beliefs of the ego/personality have been in error for this and other lifetimes. This is necessary to make progress in the journey to self-realization. Self-realized people have a single-headed and single-hearted understanding of life. This allows the balance of the mind and the body necessary to stay healthy.

"I don't believe. I must have a reason for a certain hypothesis. Either I know a thing, and then I know it - I don't need to believe it."

– Carl Jung

Relieving yourself from the chains of conditioning and programming is a process that requires a lifetime and a conscious decision to face the limiting beliefs and behaviors of others.

This certainly makes the case for staying in the moment to understand life as it unfolds. Thus, taking away past anxieties, putting pressure on current moment realities to be the same as the past, and worrying about the future of what may be, might be, could be, and shoulds where we don't have future information to decide.

"Life is a series of natural and spontaneous changes. Don't resist them; that only creates sorrow. Let reality be reality. Let things flow naturally forward in whatever way they like."

– Lao Tzu

De-Conditioning a Series of Systems

Learning to recognize our emotional responses to life events and people is beneficial. A person's affective states, such as feelings, moods, and emotional reactions, comprise the conditioned systems. One must discover subconscious motives and restore one's normal reaction to a situation to resolve emotional issues. This process uncovers the hidden treasure of emotionality by examining emotions' intensity, deep insight, content, time, and space. A positive message and bodywork are needed to eliminate negative emotions and achieve emotional freedom, clarity, and a good sense of self-worth.

For emotional integration to work, a person must deeply understand their emotions, feelings, and personal past. Learning to express one's emotions without blaming others is also crucial. Suppressing anger and sadness can lead to moods that don't integrate with emotional components. So, managing and controlling moods is also necessary to maintain balance. The process of deconditioning involves recognizing and working with a chosen response. Exploring and letting go of emotions to find emotional control brings freedom, clarity, and a healthy sense of self-worth. Differentiating between emotions and feelings addresses actions, reactions, and moods.

From Childhood to Adulthood

Many of us can relate to automatically adopting the behaviors of our parents or caregivers. We often promise ourselves that we won't do or be the things other people do that we find annoying, only to discover that we are doing those things later. People can feel shocked, angry, or even disgusted when they try to figure out why they keep repeating patterns they knew they didn't want to repeat.

One of the more exciting things is that we often don't realize we're copying the behaviors of people around us. We might not even be aware that we are imitating the same behaviors, voice tones, and words from our childhood and those we admire. Our minds are running on autopilot, following patterns deeply ingrained in us from a very young age and conditioned adults.

This is true not only for individual actions but also for relationships, job choices, and even our view of the world. We may keep doing things the way our parents or caregivers taught us, even if they are no longer helpful or good. This can make us feel like we're stuck in a rut, unable to escape the conditioning of our childhood.

When we reflect on our childhood experiences, it's important to remember that our parents and caregivers made the best use of the tools in their hands. They were likely reacting to their upbringing and conditioning without even realizing it. We don't have to blame them for the problems we're having right now. Instead, we can use this knowledge to take charge of our own lives and make choices about the kind of person we want to be.

Being aware of these habits is a crucial part of replacing them. By recognizing the programming in our subconscious mind that controls our actions, we can change them to include more powerful thoughts and routines.

We realize that our patterns make choosing authentic reactions challenging. Then, we can use techniques like emotional detachment, guided meditations, and hypnosis to change how our subconscious mind responds and adopt more positive, helpful views.

"You use hypnosis not as a cure but as a means of establishing a favorable climate in which to learn."

– Milton Erickson

We can create lives that align with our wants and values. It is possible but also necessary to start this journey of self-discovery and deliberate change to free ourselves from karmic circumstances and generational trauma.

Tools for Change

Hypnotherapy can be handy because it lets us access the subconscious mind, where our conditioning is kept. Hypnosis can help you slowly replace negative ideas with more supportive ones. NLP methods, such as reframing, anchoring, and modeling, can also be beneficial for changing behavior and thought patterns by observing positive choices in ourselves or role models.

Changes to our programming also need practice and reinforcement. New thought patterns or actions take time and repetition to become automatic. This could mean reaffirming new views daily or often or picturing what you want to happen.

Bringing in spiritual thoughts can also help the change process go more smoothly. There are many ways to do this, such as through spiritual astrology, meditation, or working with spirit guides to understand and use one's skills.

"As human beings, we do not operate behaviorally, that is, directly upon the world, but on the map or model of what we believe the world to be."

Richard Bandler & John Grinder, Pattern of Hypnotic Techniques of Milton Erickson

Freeing Ourselves from Beliefs

"Anytime you're gonna grow, you're gonna lose something. You're losing what you're hanging onto to keep safe. You're losing habits that you're comfortable with, you're losing familiarity."

– James Hillman

This highlights the profound influence of our relationships and the environment on our beliefs and behaviors. It is important to remember that we can choose and change the programming that influences our ideas and deeds.

To become our authentic selves and free ourselves from the restrictions of programming and conditioning, we need to monitor our thoughts, behaviors, actions, and reactions. We must look for automatic responses and excessive emotional reactions, which indicate an area needing processing.

Most of the time, our minds are mentally lazy and only use the smallest amount of energy needed to finish each job. Cycles of thought patterns that are never questioned or examined can cause us to act and make choices that may not align with our authentic selves, i.e., who we prefer to be.

Before changing our thinking, we must recognize the beliefs that support disharmony in our lives. Beliefs can be changed despite how deeply ingrained they are. By practicing intentionally enough, we can rewire ourselves and go beyond the limits of our old programming.

"Your beliefs become your thoughts, thoughts become your words, your words become your actions, your actions become your habits, your habits become your values, and your values become your destiny."

– Mahatma Gandhi

Confirmation Bias

"What the human being is best at doing is interpreting all new information so that their prior conclusions remain intact."

– Warren Buffet

Confirmation bias is the tendency to see new information supporting an already-held belief. It is essential to be open to different points of view and take a fluid approach to fighting confirmation bias. Additionally, we need to work on resisting the urge to support our beliefs and instead dig deeper to find the right and fair point of view that can stand the test of objectivity.

"People who accomplish a great many things are people who have freed themselves from biases. These are creative people."

– Milton Erickson

"Don't focus on winning a race just to prove yourself right; it's more important to ensure you're in the race that truly matters. Instead of constantly defending your ideas, stay open and receptive to embracing new perspectives and insights from others."

Availability Heuristics

Availability heuristics are mental shortcuts that simplify decision-making by utilizing our ability to remember information from previous experiences. To fix availability heuristics, you must take a moment before jumping to conclusions and gather correct data. In addition to what we remember, we need to do more research sometimes and think outside the box to make well-informed choices.

"The ease of recall suggests that if something is more easily recalled in your memory, you tend to think it must occur with a high probability."

– Som Bathla

Hanlon's Razor – "Negativity Bias"

Negativity bias occurs even when positive and negative events are equally intense. It makes us internalize negative experiences more intensely, causing us to worry and fixate on minor incidents.

"Misunderstandings and neglect create more confusion in this world than trickery and malice."

– Goethe, "The Sorrows of Young Werther" 1774

The Halo Effect

This is where memories induce a response instead of a thoughtful evaluation. By constantly exposing ourselves to positive stimuli, we can train our minds to think more positively.

"Life is like a camera. Just focus on what's important and capture the good times, develop from the negatives, and if things don't work out, take another shot."

– Unknown

These are a few ways to deliberately turn our conscious attention to evaluating our beliefs and habitual thinking. The idea is to gain a more positive attitude and ways of processing our lives.

Reality is influenced by our thoughts, feelings, and goals, both conscious and unconscious. When these parts work together, we create the reality we want as long as we pursue our interests, which connects us with the universe's natural rhythm.

"To be sane, we must recognize our beliefs as fiction."

– James Hillman, Healing Fiction

Visualization and Journaling

Engaging our subconscious mind through imagination is another successful strategy for changing our patterns and achieving our authentic selves.

"Jung observed that the Aboriginal people of Australia spend about two-thirds of their waking lives in some form of inner work...we modern people can scarcely get a few hours free in an entire week to devote to the inner world."

– Robert Johnson, Inner work: Using dreams and active imagination for personal growth.

We can achieve our goals and reach our full potential by considering what's possible and finding ways to make it happen. Being open-minded, not judging, and ready to investigate new possibilities can all help us improve our imagination.

Visualization is a thought that helps us create clear mental pictures of what we want and desire. It is no more difficult than picturing yesterday or tomorrow. When you visualize and work towards a goal, the subconscious mind attracts and manifests it. This is alchemy.

"Imagination is a preview of life's coming attractions."

– Albert Einstein

When we work with vision, we can change our behavior for the better and create the life we want. Our subconscious mind greatly influences this process because it generates ideas, connects different ideas, and shows us alternatives that we might not have considered before. So, relax profoundly and change.

"Thus, man of all creatures is more than a creature; he is also a creator. Man, alone can direct his success mechanism using imagination, or imaging ability."

– Maxwell Maltz

Journaling is another effective tool for change. Writing connects directly to the subconscious mind. This is where handwriting analysis comes from. I like to have clients journal their frustrations because it allows them to freely express negative emotions that are bottled up inside. Filtering out information that isn't important helps us focus on what is. This process can help us determine what patterns and protocols hinder our success and change them to better ones.

Our mental attitude and the kinds of ideas we have previously allowed to influence us significantly impact our character and self-image. By being aware of our thoughts and feelings, we can change them and build a more positive and empowering picture of ourselves.

"It's enough to decide that from now on, we won't let any bad, depressing, or unwanted thoughts enter our heads. Instead, we must immediately change these negative ideas with more positive ones. It is essential that when a negative thought comes up, we push it out of our minds right away by thinking of bright, happy, positive, and desirable ideas instead."

– William Atkinson

Yes, our personality comprises the feelings and ideas we were born with, the thoughts and ideas we are told to have, and the ideas and habits we have picked up over our lives when our Ego is quiet and inactive. Still, the ego can control its surroundings and get rid of the junk stored away from the past by waking up and using its weapon, the will.

It is crucial to talk with our emotions and thoughts and watch out for actions and ideas that attempt to avoid them. We must carefully examine our private discussions to see if they are helpful or harmful.

What are the ideas behind our negative inner dialogue? Recognize where our self-punishment comes from.

Visualization and mental images can be powerful tools for change. By picturing the desired result in our lives and working towards the goal, the subconscious mind supports us with thoughts to overcome obstacles and reach our goals.

"By willpower and perseverance, you may change the nature of your mental materials stored away in the storerooms of the Inner Consciousness, including the inherited ones, and thus render yourself practically a new person in character and nature within a reasonable time."

– William Atkinson

Chapter 8:
Empowering Inner Dialogue:
Transforming Self-Talk And Self-Image

"As you alter your self-talk, you will set up a corrective mechanism for challenging the entire structure by which you live your life. As changes in self-talk lead to changes in behavior, the external environment will usually respond to support your growth."

– Dr. Pamela E. Butler, Talking to Yourself

Our internal dialogue, or self-talk, dramatically impacts our thoughts, feelings, and actions. It includes our thoughts, words, and tone when we talk to ourselves. Our mental talk is vital to our mental health because it can make us stronger or weaker. How we communicate with ourselves can either help us get through hard times or stop us. For instance, when we fail at something, negative self-talk can creep in and push us backward by speaking our fears and doubts. But think about what would happen if we could change things. What changes would happen to our self-esteem, resilience, and drive if we knew how to use positive self-talk? By doing this, we can break free from the limits that self-doubt has put on us and reach our full potential.

"Anytime we have a negative feeling, it instantly causes a loss of 50% of our muscle strength and a narrowing of our vision both physically and mentally."

– Dr. David Hawkins. Power vs. Force

The way we communicate with ourselves has a significant impact on the body and how we feel. When we are kind to ourselves, we are more likely to feel happy, calm, and balanced. Low self-esteem, worry, and hopelessness can all happen quickly when you talk badly to yourself. This is because our brains are wired to release hormones that make us feel good or bad, depending on how we respond to our internal dialogue. When we talk to ourselves with more self-awareness, we can find limiting patterns and work to replace them.

As we improve our internal dialogue, it will start to affect our relationships. Our relationships will become more profound because we care about, understand, and help each other more. We will also be better able to deal with problems because we are more focused, driven, and firm in our resolve. Being able to talk kindly to yourself is a big part of living a happier, more meaningful life.

Two Minds Self-talk

The conscious mind is the socializing brain that evolved through evolution. It involves complex social behaviors, visual processing, and problem-solving. The subconscious mind is the mammalian brain found in all living organisms. It is responsible for coordination and fine motor control, including agility and fight-flight-freeze protection. Each mind has its task in our functioning and life.

The ego and personality are related to the conscious mind. Fundamentally, our sense of self-worth, respect, image, and self-confidence comes from the ego. The ego is self-centered and reflects our personality. Our character is housed in our conscious mind's critical, evaluating, and analytical areas.

One of life's most transforming experiences is realizing that your soul and spirit are linked in the subconscious mind. The soul is one of the main principles on which a person bases their thoughts and deeds, which come from memory. Traditionally regarded as existing apart from the physical body, living in the background, the subconscious mind always watches and records our existence. The soul's responsibility is to use all accumulated information from present and prior existence to guide us through experiences to discover our conscious perceptions that are in error. Thus, the known and unknown guidance navigates us toward experiences that bring clarity to our conditioning and programming. This guidance leads us to awaken to our authentic selves and, ultimately, enlightenment.

"It is only when the soul, using many earth-lives, begins to see the worthlessness and illusory nature of earthly desires, that it begins to become attracted by the things of the life of its higher nature, and, escaping the flowing currents of earthly re-birth, it rises above them and is carried to higher spheres."

– The Complete Works of William Walker Atkinson Ego vs Soul: Two different entities.

Simplified, your ego, conscious mind, is your mask or image of yourself; your soul is your spirit, essence, and authentic self is embedded in the subconscious mind. Why do we allow the ego mind to decide what is real? This is a fundamental way we choose our beliefs depending on our experiences and realities. We conceive a meaning for the world we create. The problem with that? The ego mind survives by upholding one's viewpoint at the expense of others. This becomes a moral judgment of the actions of others while defending our actions and behaviors. Our lifetime(s) of judgments, conclusions, and decisions have bound us to a personalized reality, hiding the actual reality only experienced now.

"The ego is constantly judging everything and everyone, including itself and its behavior. This judging aims to survive by being right, although not necessarily responsible. The ego defends itself against other egos by considering itself right and making others wrong, by validating its own opinion and position and invalidating the opinions and positions of others."

– Luke Rinehart, The Book of EST

Negative Self-Talk

We can now understand where negative thoughts originate. The need to survive by being right. These beliefs and thoughts have a massive impact on our lives. This means that we have the power to stop ourselves from reaching our full potential. We are responsible for our thoughts and actions. What we think and believe is what we create.

"If you allow experiences of the past to overshadow your future, you are ensuring there is no future in your life, just recycling the past."

– Sadhguru

The thoughts and dialogue we have with ourselves, whether positive or negative, significantly impact our health, motivation, and sense of self-worth. As long as we keep reminding ourselves of our skills, we are more likely to push ourselves to follow our guidance and reach our goals. When we think about our flaws and question ourselves, we are more likely to hold back and play it safe, risking greater possibilities.

"What would you attempt to do if you knew you could not fail?"

– Unknown

Positive Self-Talk

Positive self-talk is a powerful tool for overcoming difficulties and achieving our goals. Positive self-talk, like "I can do it" or "I'm capable," can help us overcome problems, strengthen, and develop a growth mindset. We can keep going when things get tough and keep our drive, focus, and commitment to our goals. Through positive self-talk, we can overcome our self-doubt and limits and reach our full potential. We must choose whether to be our best friend or worst enemy. We must remember that soul guidance is always present. That support system is positive self-talk and belief in ourselves. We are where we are supposed to be at any given moment and have the tools to succeed, or we would not be in that moment.

"Psychological stress resides neither in the person nor in the situation. It depends on the transaction between the two. It comes from how a person assesses the situation they are currently in and the efforts they exert to adapt to it. The effect of the situation on our mood and our health depends on its frequency and intensity."

– R.S. Lazarus

Close your eyes and think of something you would like to accomplish. As you picture it being done, say aloud, "No matter how hard it is, I can do it. " Now, scan your body. Notice how you feel. Are you feeling successful?

The natural progression of beliefs follows a pattern. Programming and conditioning create belief; belief creates attitudes; attitudes create feelings; feelings determine actions; actions create results, and results create karma.

It is often said that self-talk can significantly impact your confidence. Whether positive or negative, it can affect what and how you feel differently. So, it is indeed crucial to practice positive self-talk. After all, we cannot deny the fact that negativity can destroy even the slightest hope. Evaluating how and why we respond the way we do becomes very important. In other words, we must sort through our mental conversations at any given moment and decide if they are conditioned responses from past experiences or programmed responses that are or are not our best choices.

Remember, if the conscious mind is confused and coincides with emotion, the subconscious will immediately respond with a default action or re-action, even freeze, since it will be evaluated as a threat. That response will protect you and is conditioned from a similar experience in the past. And that response happens in 2 milliseconds, faster than the 55 milliseconds it takes the conscious mind to respond. This can easily lead to self-sabotage. You are now living in and responding to the past instead of staying present in the moment and responding with a conscious choice.

Self-talk of the Two Minds

Intrinsic Self (Self-realized) vs. Imposed Self (Conditioned)

We all have an innate conscience that is a compass recognized as an inner voice of guidance, a still small voice, an intuitive feeling—our co-creative self. The *Authentic, intrinsic self* encompasses our intuition, originality, sincerity, freedom, and fun. Our angels, guides, and teachers are always present and support us in becoming our Universal Creator selves. It's our Soul. To live with confidence and guidance, you listen to your self-talk and gut instinct, a unique voice in your mind. One step in the right direction is becoming aware of what thought produces the best feeling. This will help you spot harmful internal dialogue patterns and slowly change them to ones that are more caring and helpful.

A conditioned or patterned response does not always fit the current moment since it is the voice of the conscious mind that uses the language of our programmers. This voice may or may not fit who we choose to be while using the reason and logic of others and present and past life experiences. A self that we and others impose on us. Throughout our lives, we develop what is commonly called the *'Enforcer Self,'* also known as the 'Conditioned Self' or the 'Ego Self,' as we interact with the world around us. Our opinions about what is right and wrong, 'good enough,' and "not good enough," are shaped by our parents, instructors, and society. Our behavior and self-judgment are influenced by external factors, which shape internal norms.

The challenge is that the conflict between our *"Authentic Self"* and our *"Enforcer Self"* is crucial as we face life's difficulties. We use the past or fears of the future in present life, NOW, circumstances where the choice does not align with our authentic decisions and values.

The Authentic/Soul Self

It's fascinating to think about how our conditioning can shape us, but beneath all that lies our true essence – 'the *Authentic Self*,' also known as the 'Soul Self.' It tells us that you're not one to let others' expectations sway you. It's a fundamental part of your identity. It symbolizes your unique aspirations, the power that lies within you, and your true essence.

The *Authentic Self* is characterized by the following:

Intuition: When we discuss intuition, we refer to that inner understanding and gut feeling that guides us in the right direction. Feelings and emotions are the only truths. Intuition is the ability to acquire knowledge without interference or using reason. Intuit comes from the Latin 'intueri,' often roughly translated as 'to look inside' or 'to contemplate.'

Creativity encompasses a boundless wellspring of ideas, passions, and abilities. *"Man has no choice other than to use his creative power. His thought will always be creative, whether he knows it or not. The creativity of man's thought has nothing to do with his will or belief; it is here just as nature is. It is the use of a creative power that man has control over, not the thing itself."*

– Ernest Holmes, The Science of Mind

Authenticity is about expressing yourself genuinely and living your life based on your values. *"Divine love is not judgment or denial of self-truths. The Divine Law is honoring harmony that comes from a peaceful mind, an open heart, a true tongue, a light step, a forgiving nature, and a love of all living creatures."* – Jamie Sams and David Carson, Medicine Cards, Native American

Empowerment: Having the confidence to take control of your life and pursue your aspirations is what we call empowerment. *"You can use everything that happens in your life as a process of empowerment or to entangle yourself."*

– Sadhguru

Joy is the beautiful feeling that comes from living authentically, bringing a sense of satisfaction and fulfillment. Our perspective on life shifts when we take the time to cultivate our inner selves. We align our decisions with our personal goals, rely on our instincts, and unleash our creative power. As a result, we experience a greater sense of purpose, fulfillment, and connection to ourselves and the world around us.

The Judge/Enforcer Self

The *Enforcer Self* comes in many shapes and sizes depending on social, familial, conditioning, and programming. It is marked by harsh criticism, unrealistic standards, low faith in one's abilities, and a lack of self-worth. Our inner critic stands ready to protect us from failure. It's always finding something wrong with us and telling us we're not good enough, the challenge is too big, or we're not smart enough.

The enforcer self is the Judge. It's the critical, fault-finding, blaming self-talk with the penalties to go along with it. The Judge has its helpers. There are four main ways in which the enforcer self can manifest:

The Evaluator/Critic: This voice tends to be critical, always looking for flaws and faults. Perfectionism is crucial for its survival, and it often leaves us feeling inadequate.

The Inner Charioteer: This voice always pushes us with high expectations and demands that can be overwhelming. It often surpasses our limits and eventually causes burnout.

The Doubting Thomas: This voice dampens our enthusiasm and instills doubt, making us hesitant to take risks or pursue our goals, regardless of our motivations.

The Programmers: This voice distorts our sense of reality by introducing biases and assumptions, making it challenging to think clearly and make decisions.

Dealing with the constant chatter of the enforcer Self can be challenging at times. Feeling down on oneself, constantly questioning abilities, and always feeling like one is not measuring up are all possible results of this situation. Negativity can take a toll on our mental and emotional well-being. It can make it harder for us to be true to ourselves, face challenges head-on, and form meaningful connections with others.

Everyone has a driver or *"pusher,"* which calls us to please others, be perfect, hurry up, try harder, and be strong. These are the unconscious pushers, and they come from the programming received in early life. Knowing the voice of the pusher can enhance your well-being and improve your relationships, effectiveness, communication, and creativity.

The *"Doubting Thomas"* is part of the human personality. These come as warnings learned very early once we become mobile: "Don't touch the stove; it's hot." "Don't touch" is the authority voice, while "It's hot" is the concerned voice for our welfare. Naturally, our heritage's doubts, insecurities, and values are passed down until our dialogue and values become the truths and beliefs of our lives.

We often make assumptions about everything we need clarification on. This is the *"Confusers."* Confusions are merely two different things – the one you are starting to learn and the one you cannot understand. Personal whim beliefs, blaming self and others, tunnel vision, overgeneralization, and magnifying events or situations are the ways of thinking and perceiving that prevent us from totally experiencing what the world is. Confusers deter us from experiencing the world as it is.

We became predictors about the outcome even when we did not take a single step towards that outcome. How will we know? We categorize and conclude the people and other things around us based on our perceptions. We can help avoid confusion by accepting things as they are and believing in ourselves rather than our opinions.

"Life is a series of natural and spontaneous changes. Don't resist them; that only creates sorrow. Let reality be reality. Let things flow naturally forward in whatever way they like."

– Lao Tzu

Maintaining Positive Self-Talk

Our minds are constantly filled with thoughts, emotions, and wants that vie for our attention. There are moments of encouragement and support within this world, yet they are often overshadowed by a prevailing critical voice that plants doubt and amplifies fears. The voice you hear is the product of cultural conditioning and past experiences.

We must practice being aware of the moment to slow down the Enforcer Self. You clear your mind and visualize the result. Start working toward the goal. The subconscious mind knows how to accomplish the vision. Trust the process. St. Germain called this "alchemy."

All negative self-talk comes from memory and forms a picture or image of something out of your past. Immediately remember a happy time and good memory, hold that memory in place for three deep breaths, and watch the old memory fade away. Make a fist and feel the feelings of happiness.

Getting in touch with our bodies is crucial to access our natural knowledge and power. It's essential to enjoy our wins, no matter how small, because it makes us feel better about ourselves, keeps us motivated, and helps us reach our ultimate goals. Self-kindness is also very important because it allows us to be as understanding, sympathetic, and kind to ourselves as we would be to a close friend.

Most people are subjective toward themselves and objective toward others, but the task is to be objective to ourselves and subjective toward others.

"Self-talk" is a necessary ingredient, like stripping away the layers of onion from our character, which are molded by the actions, thoughts, beliefs, and fears of others. These are the tools of the conscious mind and the subconscious programmed into our emotional nature. They drive the memories of response before we have time to decide when dealing with the current presentation of experience.

As we are educated and mature with healthy self-esteem, we can question the truth and beliefs we grow up with, allowing us to form our realities as we begin living through trial and error. But without a perfect environment, we take on the fears, anxieties, and human characteristics that can challenge us in life. Now, the " do nots" of authority ring in our heads as if we've never left the parental fold.

Our minds are constantly filled with thoughts, emotions, and wants that vie for our attention. There are moments of encouragement and support within this world, yet they are often overshadowed by a prevailing critical voice that plants doubt and amplifies fears. The voice you hear is the product of cultural conditioning and past experiences.

"The attractions are not innate to the world but reflect projected values and the expectation of the payoffs of ego satisfaction. Joy stems from

within and is not dependent on externals. Pleasure is associated with what is valued and esteemed. Much of projected value arises from imagination, and values reflect desires. In reality, nothing is more valuable than anything else other than spiritual fulfillment."

– Dr. David Hawkins, Along the Path to Enlightenment

Managing Negative Self-Talk

Transitioning from a constantly criticized self to nurturing your inner voice is a journey. Here are a few steps you can take to develop your genuine voice and handle any negativity you may be experiencing:

Become Aware: The initial step is to be aware of the ongoing dialogue within your mind. Take a moment to be mindful of the thoughts and emotions you're experiencing throughout the day. Pay close attention to what happens when the Enforcer, the Pusher, or the Doubting Thomas takes charge.

Challenge Your Thoughts: Let's challenge the notion that negativity represents the ultimate truth. It's worth considering the validity of critical thoughts and finding ways to reframe them more positively. When you think, you can only believe in evaluating terms, meaning you are thinking in terms of duality where the ego mind is dominant. Likewise, when you feel you are experiencing a relationship and connectedness, The Higher mind and High Heart dominate. *"Stop thinking and end your problems."*

– Lao Tzu

Embrace Mindfulness: This can bring a sense of calmness to the mind and create space for the true self to shine through. Practices like meditation and mindful breathing are great examples of techniques that can be used. *"You should meditate for twenty minutes daily – unless you're too busy. Then it would be best if you sat for an hour."*

– Zen proverb

Practicing Gratitude: This can help you cultivate a more positive outlook and break free from negativity. It's helpful to shift your focus towards the positive aspects of your life. *"If the interest is detached from the plane of sense gratification, if there is a constant effort to fix the mind on the attainment of the highest ideal, the result will be that the past Karma will find no basis in which to inhere on the physical plane."*

– The Theosophy Society

Connect with Your Body: Participating in physical activities and incorporating practices like yoga can help you feel more present and reconnect with your inner wisdom. Every thought, every reverberation you create on the level of the mind changes the chemistry in your body. Your muscles lose fifty percent of strength with a negative thought. Try it. Test your strength when thinking positive thoughts and then opposing thoughts.

Embrace Positive Affirmations: Acknowledging and appreciating your strengths and accomplishments is essential. By consistently recognizing and affirming your positive qualities, you can counteract negativity and boost your self-confidence. So, don't hesitate to embrace self-praise.

Explore and Nurture Your Interests: Embrace your authentic self and find fulfillment in activities that bring you happiness and allow your creativity to flourish. *"Don't think. Thinking is the enemy of creativity. It's self-conscious, and anything self-conscious is lousy. You can't try to do things. It would be best if you did things."*

– Ray Bradbury

Celebrate the Triumph of Little Things: Regardless of how small your achievements may seem, it's essential to recognize them. When this happens, it's great to see positive behaviors being rewarded and motivation being boosted. The subconscious mind is motivated by rewards.

Summary: Contact trusted friends, family members, or a mental health professional to seek support and discuss your experience. They can provide objectivity, encouragement, and a fresh perspective. Self-compassion is all about treating yourself with the same love and understanding you would give to a close friend. This is a friendly reminder to approach your journey with patience and kindness as you progress. It's essential to understand the importance of setting boundaries and prioritizing self-care. Saying *"no"* when necessary is a vital part of this process. It helps conserve energy and build a strong connection with your inner self. Explore your awareness. Why not spend a little while reflecting on yourself and delving into your thoughts? Exploring personal growth courses, therapy, and journaling can help you better understand your thoughts, feelings, and values.

Cultivate a Strong Connection with Spirit

Yes, you read it right. You can cultivate a connection with the Spirit. But how can you connect with your spirit so that it can naturally become a dominant force in your life? To help you maximize flow, joy, and peace in your life, here are crucial keys to get you started:

Live in the Present—If you truly live in the present moment, you have greater access to your Spirit. Feelings are the gateway to communication for most. When you focus on the past (emotions), pain, turmoil, and regret can overtake you and cut your connection with your Spirit.

Moreover, when you focus on the future, you are often distracted by fear, worry, and hope, which will starve your energy from creating your present or visualizing your future. Now, in the present moment, you can find joy, peace, and a genuine connection with your Spirit.

Choose High Vibrations—Use peace, love, joy, generosity, appreciation, and more good feelings in your self-talk to strengthen your connection with your Spirit and deflate the barriers of the ego. When manifesting abundance, always focus on good feelings.

Take Responsibility for Conscious Choices—The ego likes playing "victim," which leads to the belief that you are not powerful or have any choice. Whatever the situation, a responsible and powerful choice will always be available. Do not be a victim and choose to make a conscious choice.

Stop Overthinking—This is tough. Human minds are often ego-dominated and run nonstop. Most of us may assume that thinking is intelligent, but when the ego takes over, we tend to overthink. Different thinking appears when our minds are still and enlivens our connection with our spirit. A way to do this is to focus on anything for ten seconds or close your eyes and focus on breathing deeply ten times.

Humility—The ego is all about criticizing, being right, judging, etc. When you become humble, you will release the grip of your ego faster. You will become accepting of yourself and continue to grow and evolve.

"The conscious use of spiritual power is the finest of arts because it is deeply felt...its whole thought is based on the intimate relationship of the Spirit with everything that is. It is scientific in that it deals with law and order.... the effective practitioner in this science has the will to try, the courage to attempt, and the faith to believe in himself because he has confidence in the Law of Good. The simplicity of this conviction is enhanced when he realizes he has nothing to change outside himself."

– Ernest Holmes, "The Science of Mind"

Self-Image

"We suffer more in our imagination than in reality."

- Seneca

A person's self-image is how they see themselves on the inside. Identity is complex and multidimensional, including more than just how someone looks. It includes their character, skills, and values as well. We can't say enough about how important a person's self-image is for their mental health, behavior, and sense of self-worth.

The things we do and how we connect with our families as children begin the process of shaping our self-image. Our biological and cultural parents significantly impact how we form our essential self-image. Loving and supportive situations are more likely to help people build good self-images.

The problems we must solve in our lives are planned by the rules of karmic necessity to discover who we are: co-creators. Accepting our true selves and living our lives according to our choices provides the opportunity for growth and a greater sense of self-awareness. Societal and national norms affect a person's self-image. Our ideals of success, appearance, and behavior can shape our self-perception as we strive for social acceptance. This is about maintaining a positive self-perception of physical characteristics, such as attractiveness, physical skills, and body image. How someone feels about themselves in this area can significantly impact their self-worth. Friends, social networks, and professional relationships affect a person's self-image as they age. The influence of one's peer group on one's self-image and feeling of acceptance and belonging is not always positive.

"You don't have to change who you are for anyone: if you are your regular, authentic, confident self, then you can push to do whatever you want."

– Maya Angelou

Unfortunately, a group can decide how we feel about things and what others say. If we look to the outside world to define us, others can boost and lower a person's sense of self-worth and self-image with praise, success, criticism, rejection, and put-downs. Why look outside for personal definition? Being proud of your accomplishments and reaching your goals can help you feel better about yourself.

Your perfect self is the best version of yourself you feel you should be, along with your success goals, values, and even quirky personality traits. The difference between who someone is and who they think they should be could affect their drive and sense of self-worth. Self-esteem is the part of your self-image that judges you. People can see their sense of value and self-worth in it. A good self-image is often linked to high self-esteem. A lousy self-image and lack of confidence could also come from failures and disappointments. People who have mental health problems like depression and worry often have low self-esteem. If you think well of yourself, you're more likely to be mentally stable, driven, and successful. Self-esteem makes people stronger, happier, healthier, and mentally stable. It also strengthens connections and makes people more resilient.

"Thinking is difficult. That's why most people judge."

– Carl Jung

Mindfulness and self-reflection, positive self-talk and affirmations, setting attainable goals, surrounding oneself with helpful people, and making good lifestyle choices are all things that can help improve one's self-image. Understanding oneself and working on having a good self-image can help people live whole and healthy lives.

Final Duality: Feminine-Masculine Self

"We must awaken to our female archetype or goddess figures; we must ask ourselves repeatedly what our real needs are, experience them, validate them, and restructure our lives so that we may meet them as fully as possible."

– Tracy Marks, Astrologer, Psychotherapist, The Astrology of Self-Discovery

Balancing feminine and masculine energies within oneself is essential for holistic well-being. Embracing feminine energy allows for a more intuitive, compassionate, and connected life, complementing masculine energy's action-oriented and goal-driven nature. Integrating both can lead to a more harmonious and fulfilled existence, where one can be both nurturing and assertive, intuitive and logical.

In a broader sense, *giving* is an action of our divine masculine, and *receiving* is an action of our sacred feminine. A balance of both energies is when we feel harmonious within. Where the masculine is about the will, the feminine receives the masculine's impressions and works on producing new ideas, thoughts, concepts, and all works of imagination to create or birth the masculine's goal.

THE TRAITS OF FEMININE ENERGY

Feminine energy encompasses qualities such as nurturing, intuition, and receptivity. It complements masculine energy, creating a balanced and harmonious existence. Here are some critical aspects of feminine power:

1. Nurturing and Compassion: Feminine energy is deeply caring and empathetic, focusing on the well-being and support of others. Relate to others by listening, sharing, and nurturing.

2. Intuition and Inner Knowing emphasize inner wisdom, intuition, and a deep connection to feelings and emotions. They magnetically attract and see the big picture.

3. Receptivity and Flow: Feminine energy is open, adaptable, and responsive. It values the ability to go with the flow rather than forcing outcomes. It holds the space for projects to develop at their natural pace.

4. Creativity and Expression: Feminine creativity enjoys the creation process independent of the results. It has artistic expression and the ability to birth new ideas and projects.

5. Collaboration and Community: Feminine energy fosters connection, cooperation, and building relationships, valuing collective well-being over individual achievement. Works with others to create community.

6. Healing and Transformation: This energy is strongly linked to healing, growth, and transformation, often working through cycles and phases. With weak feminine energy, masculine energy functions without order, restraint, or reason, resulting in utter chaos. They stay in wild goose chase mode.

THE TRAITS OF MASCULINE ENERGY

Masculine energy is often associated with assertiveness, strength, logic, and leadership. It complements feminine energy associated with nurturing, intuition, and receptivity. Here are some critical aspects of masculine energy:

1. Action-oriented: Masculine energy is about acting, making decisions, and moving forward. It embodies the principle of doing and achieving, and it leads to projects.

2. Strength and Courage: This energy is often linked with physical and emotional strength and the courage to face challenges and take risks. Make the decisions along the way towards progress.

3. Logic and Reasoning: Masculine energy favors rational thinking, analysis, and problem-solving. It values structure, order, and clarity—continuous problem-solving.

4. Independence: It promotes self-reliance, autonomy, and the ability to stand alone and be self-sufficient. It involves living a structured and planned life.

5. Goal-Driven: Setting and achieving goals, ambition, and focusing on outcomes is central to masculine energy. Career-focused and have disciplined goals.

6. Protection and Provision: Traditionally, masculine energy includes the roles of protector and provider, ensuring the safety and well-being of others. It also involves compartmentalizing emotions and not allowing emotions to overshadow logic.

With weak masculine energy, then the feminine will always remain in the realm of imagination without taking action to create concrete results, leading to complacency and stagnation.

This is the desired relationship between the conscious mind and the subconscious mind. The conscious mind sets a goal or will for something, while the subconscious works to bring that thing forth. The magic is to visualize the goal (feminine) and then work towards it daily, one day at a time (masculine).

~∞

Chapter 9:
Hypnosis And Healing

"Healing in the present moment involves resolving the unfinished business of the past, which continues to influence a person in the present moment. The residual mental, emotional, physical, and spiritual energy of past events contaminates the present experience. Resolving the removal of burdensome energies is the goal of any healing approach. Then a person can live more fully in the present and fulfill more completely the details of the life plan."

– William J Baldwin, Spirit Releasement Therapy

Redefining Healing in the Coming Age

Many ways of healing have been used throughout history. The root word of 'healing' is *hale*, or *"to make whole."* It is impossible to separate what is mental from the physical or spiritual, yet our language does not offer concepts to understand these connections best. Some healing techniques have been around for thousands of years, while others have only been around for a few hundred.

The point of healing is to bring the mind, body, and soul into balance and harmony. The key here is that something in the mind and body was out of balance and supported the illness or disease. When our family dynamics, such as epigenetics, are at fault or when a stable change of cell function occurs without modifications to the DNA sequence, this does not mean we give up on being healthy. This means that our challenge is to fight against our heritage and programming. Just because one is prone to heart disease, one's responsibility is to maintain a diet that controls cardiovascular disease.

Psychological factors can also affect illness, disease, or an inharmonious life. Even our spiritual life can be at the core of our problems. We are all familiar with the saying "body-mind-spirit" as a common healing strategy. Problems can manifest on any one of these levels.

"What is held in the mind tends to manifest...including unconscious beliefs."

– Dr. David Hawkins

The modern way to identify a disorder is to label a problem. This creates ownership of a problem in many circumstances, such as "my pain," "my fear," and even "my anxiety." Once named, it is easy to believe in the disability of a diagnosed condition and more challenging to get rid of the conflict. What makes it worse is that each comes with its medication. This makes it difficult to convince people in some cases, they can heal themselves. Now, instead of taking any responsibility for self-healing, the reliance on drugs supports "my problem." What is the belief that supports the condition? Medication may sometimes be a necessity, but are there natural remedies? Where do body, mind, and soul fit in to find balance in all parts of oneself?

"Our perception of the body must shift from: "I am the body" to "I have a body"...here is where the mind is experiencing the body."

– Dr. David Hawkins

When you have a body, you focus on repair instead of the problem. Multiple avenues for healing can then be explored, and in some cases, the proper remedy can be found. My experience of having a heart attack allowed me to evaluate my lifestyle, diet, and physical health. Given the standard medication, even after making corrections, I had another heart attack two years later, which is what happens in a high percentage of first events. Again, I was told that my natural healing methods were a bunch of hooey, even after achieving great lab results. So, I turned to a concierge doctor who taught me all the necessary labs needing adjustments and how to get them normal. As I write this, my second event was eight years ago, and my last cardiologist appointment claimed my labs were perfect and I didn't need to return.

"The body is the reflection of the spirit in its physical expression, and its problems are the dramatization of the struggles of the spirit that gives it life."

– Dr. David Hawkins, Power vs. Force

There are Many Systems of Healing

Some systems have existed for many thousands of years. Each method has its treatments, assumptions, and a model for naming and treating various problems. Integrating the role of Allopathic, Behavioral, and Transpersonal Medicine systems creates a soul/mind/body healing system. This idea is becoming increasingly acceptable, an understood concept transcending a one-size-fits-all healing system.

> *"The person must find the courage to direct his attention to the phenomena of illness. His illness itself must no longer seem to him contemptible. Still, it must become an enemy worthy of his mettle, a piece of his personality with solid grounds for its existence and from which things of value for his future life must be derived. The way is thus paved for the reconciliation with the repressed material, which is coming to expression in his symptoms, while at the same time, a place is found for a certain tolerance for the state of being ill."*

> – Sigmund Freud

Allopathic medicine

Allopathic medicine, also known as conventional or Western medicine, is a system of medical practice that aims to combat disease by using remedies such as drugs or surgery, which produce effects different from those caused by the disease being treated. This approach contrasts with other medical systems like homeopathy, which might use substances that cause similar symptoms to treat diseases.

Our medical community relies on scientific research and evidence to determine the effectiveness of treatments. The focus is on diagnosing diseases and conditions through tests and procedures, followed by treatments to cure or manage symptoms. This includes a wide range of specialties and subspecialties, each focusing on a specific aspect of health or type of disease.

Medications are used to treat, manage, or prevent diseases. This includes everything from antibiotics to chemotherapy drugs. The importance of vaccinations, screenings, and lifestyle changes to prevent diseases is emphasized. Surgery sometimes involves removing, repairing, or replacing diseased tissues or organs.

"Any doctor will admit that any drug can have side effects and that writing a prescription involves weighing the potential benefits against the risks."

— Mark Udall

Allopathic medicine has successfully treated acute conditions, infections, and emergencies. It often incorporates advancements in technology and research to improve patient care continually. However, it may be complemented by other approaches, such as holistic or integrative medicine, to address aspects of health and well-being that go beyond physical symptoms.

Behavioral medicine

People have been trying to become more self-aware for a very long time. Today, mental medicine, which is only about a hundred and twenty years old, is based on the ideas of Sigmund Freud. Behavioral medicine is the study of how to use knowledge from social, behavioral, psychological, and biological fields to help people who are healthy or sick. "Behavioral Medicine" is a branch of science based on the idea that our actions affect our physical and mental health. This is where you can find psychologists, psychiatrists, and other mental health professionals who work with behavior, like hypnotherapists. Physiology, pharmacology, nutrition, hormones, neuroanatomy, and immunology are some of them. Hypnosis is another one. Behavioral medicine tries to help and encourage the healing of the mind's role in our health and actions. It focuses on the mind and healing. This is the idea that any disturbance or imbalance that leads to illness or sabotaging behavior affects body-mind function. Behavioral medicine has gained legitimacy primarily because the field has established an academic research base with conservative claims, having cooperated with and deferred to allopathic medicine.

"It is an odd thing, owing life to pills, one's quirks and tenacities, and this unique, strange, and ultimately profound relationship called psychotherapy."

– Kay Redfield Jamison

Transpersonal medicine

The third healing system defines some of *the oldest methods known to man,* including an ever-increasing awareness by the masses, and the other two systems used are that of Transpersonal Medicine. This healing system looks beyond the development and expression of the self to the more significant, more cosmic, global, and spiritual person of the human community. The principle of transpersonal medicine is that power in sources beyond the self ordinarily considered consensual reality can be drawn upon and used to help heal ourselves and others. The system is one of utilizing the unseen energy body and using the beyond self-powers to effect healing. One of the underlying assumptions of transpersonal medicine is that "something" is usually invisible, transferred among and between individuals, from God, or from other living and non-living objects that serve in a healing capacity. The things we typically call "energy," "prayer," "visions," "dreams," and so on. Transpersonal medicine, as a concept and practice, has re-emerged because of two significant trends:

1. The frustration with the allopathic model of medicine which has tried unsuccessfully to control the natural order by attempting to create a deathless or disease-free society.

2. *"The lack of attention and respect given to the emotional and spiritual needs of people who are ill."* (Lawlis, G.F., Transpersonal Medicine: A New Approach to Healing Body-Mind-Spirit, 1996)

The acupuncture system, TCM or Traditional Chinese Medicine, is part of a 20,000-year-old healing procedure gaining greater appeal and acceptance. But this system also includes prayer, Shamanism, and faith healing and uses ritual, music, ceremony, dream work, and many other modalities that bring healing and balance into our lives. Also included in this system are Reiki, QiGong, Chakra Balancing, Vibrational healing, energy healing of many types, and so on. All are having and gaining respect and with many valid results. And, of course, Hypnosis.

"The mind controls so much of the body. We are much more than flesh and blood; we are complex systems. Patients do better when they have faith that they will do better. That's why I always tell my patients and their families not to neglect their prayers. There's nobody I don't say that to."

– Ben Carson, MD

Integrative medicine is a new way of healing that is still in its early stages. This method tries to create a space for healing the soul, mind, and body or a chance for healing the whole person. As people learn to take charge of their health, they also know they have the power and tools to fix themselves mentally. This method shows how important it is to answer with skill and give people the tools to be involved in their healing.

The relationship between the patient and practitioner is collaborative. Practitioners take time to understand the patient's lifestyle, beliefs, and preferences. This approach emphasizes integrating all aspects of a person's well-being, including physical, emotional, mental, social, spiritual, and environmental factors.

We combine conventional medical treatments with evidence-based complementary therapies, such as acupuncture, nutrition, herbal medicine, chiropractic care, and mind-body practices. This approach to healing focuses on preventive care and promotes healthy lifestyle choices to prevent illness, emphasizing the body's innate capacity for healing.

Common Modalities Used in the Integrative Approach:

1. Mind-Body Practices:
    o   Meditation and Mindfulness
    o   Yoga and Tai Chi
    o   Hypnotherapy and Guided Imagery
    o   Stress Management Techniques

2. Nutritional and Herbal Medicine:
    o   Nutritional Supplements and Dietary Plans
    o   Herbal Therapies and Phytotherapy

3. Manipulative and Body-Based Therapies:
   o Chiropractic and Osteopathic Manipulation
   o Massage Therapy

4. Energy-Based Therapies:
   o Reiki and Healing Touch
   o Acupuncture and Acupressure

5. Traditional and Alternative Medicine:
   o Traditional Chinese Medicine (TCM)
   o Ayurveda
   o Naturopathy

Integrative Medicine is particularly useful in managing chronic conditions, enhancing recovery from illness, and promoting overall wellness. It aligns well with your interest in holistic healing and spiritual coaching. Integrative medicine incorporates various therapeutic approaches, including traditional knowledge and allopathic, behavioral, and spiritual insights, to help individuals achieve a balanced state of health.

What can hypnosis do?

Hypnotic healing has the power to change people's lives. Hypnosis is a powerful way to heal and grow because it lets us reach our subconscious and change habits, beliefs, and experiences that aren't helping us and could hurt our minds and bodies. Hypnotists can help their clients find peace and mending by using suggestions, therapy, visualization, and rituals to help them change their negative thoughts and actions.

Some of the best things about hypnosis are that it can help you understand your faith and connect with a higher power. This could significantly affect a person's mind, making them feel better and preventing illness. Regression work is beneficial for finding and rethinking events from the past that may be causing unwanted patterns of behavior in the present.

Hypnosis focuses on the creative power of the mind, which directly affects the process of making things happen. People can picture the changes they want to see and make them happen to improve their health, exercise, and quality of life in general.

One of the best things about trance healing is that it gives people control over their health and well-being. You can actively participate in your healing if you talk to your subconscious or "doctor within," Use what you learn to make choices that lead to our best health, harmony, and balance.

"Each patient carries his own doctor inside him. They come to us not knowing that truth. We are at our best when we give the doctor who resides within each patient a chance to go to work."

– Albert Schweitzer

Hypnosis is a natural condition of focused attention, increased suggestibility, and deep relaxation. It is usually brought about by verbal prompts and suggestions, helping a person to avoid the critical conscious mind and reach the subconscious mind more directly. In this state, people are generally more receptive to positive suggestions, therapeutic methods, or exploring more profound aspects of their thoughts, feelings, or memories. Hypnosis is often used for things like reducing stress, changing behavior, managing pain, and discovering subconscious patterns or beliefs. Despite common misunderstandings, hypnosis does not mean losing control or going unconscious; instead, the person remains aware and can still make choices during the process.

Simply put, the subconscious mind becomes highly responsive to suggestions to change conditioning, programming patterns, and conflicts in life. The critical analytical conscious mind relaxes and allows the more powerful subconscious mind to present suggestions as a new alternative to ways of viewing experiences, including habits and behaviors. The new options offered in hypnotic suggestions extend into the waking conscious mind and become the latest choice of response now supported by the subconscious mind.

"Physical phenomena also shift under the influence of hypnosis."

– Dr. David Hawkins

When asked what hypnosis is, I often tell clients that we go in and out of hypnosis all day long. Hypnosis is when the conscious mind is no longer analyzing, evaluating, or judging but in a state of observing. It's more like driving down the road and missing a turn. Where are we? When daydreaming, watching television, listening to the radio, or even reading where, we are more likely not thinking and analyzing. It's the state just before falling asleep where relaxation is more important than thinking.

The language of the subconscious mind uses few words, if any. It is more visual or kinesthetic (five significant senses, including muscle memory). It activates an action using stories, pictures, experiences, or feelings.

There are many misperceptions about hypnosis brought on by vampire movies and pocket-watch demonstrations, along with the misunderstanding of what's happening in stage hypnosis where there is compliance on the part of individuals who choose to participate in the show. There is never a loss of consciousness. You don't surrender your will; you will not divulge secrets nor ever get stuck in hypnosis. Another fact is that the wiser you are, the easier it is to allow the hypnotic state.

One of the many mysterious things about hypnosis is how it works. Even though there is much research on the subject, experts still struggle to agree on a clear definition of the trance experience. Hypnosis is helpful with illness on mental, physical, and spiritual levels. Among the most common reasons why hypnosis is used are dental procedures, headaches, childbirth, and pain.

A feeling of "numbness" across the body is one of the fantastic things that can happen when you are in a hypnotic trance. A skilled therapist can make any part of the body experience numbness, which is paramount to helping people manage pain.

"You use hypnosis not as a cure but as a means of establishing a favorable climate in which to learn."

– Milton Erickson

It is in the body's nature to heal itself. This complicated process happens independently, but hypnotic methods can speed up and improve it. If you tell your inner mind to do so, some parts of your body will get more of its natural resources. For instance, if you get burned, your body will start the repair process, which might take seven days to finish. Using hypnosis can speed up this process and has been shown to cut the healing time in half. The healing process is quickened whenever the focus is not on the pain.

"The subconscious mind communicates with intent. Intent is the language of doing or being within our mind."

– Larry Garrett, Hypnotist

Hypnosis is highly beneficial for relieving pain. How well this method works depends on several factors, like how open and ready the subject is to use it, how skilled the hypnotherapist is, and how significant the problem is. Because hypnosis has no adverse side effects, it can be advantageous to try along with self-hypnosis.

"There is no coming to consciousness without pain. People will do anything, no matter how absurd, to avoid facing their Soul. One does not become enlightened by imagining figures of light, but by making the darkness conscious."

– Carl Jung

Hypnosis: Medicine or Magic

Hypnosis is an old technique with a long history, dating upwards of three thousand years. In old India, people who were sick would go to sleep centers to get better. This is where hypnosis began. People in these temples would use hypnotic suggestions to put people into a trance-like state as part of their religious and healing practices. It wasn't just an Indian thing; people in ancient Greece and Egypt did the same thing. The body heals much faster in a profoundly relaxed or trance state.

Avicenna, a Persian physician (980–1037), played a key role in the emergence of hypnosis as a separate field. He was the first person to notice that hypnosis is a separate mental state from sleep that can be made and used for therapeutic purposes. In 1027, he wrote "The Book of Healing," which revealed the link between the mind and body and how hypnosis could change it. He listed the five senses, talked about many mental diseases, and explained why people lose their memories, have seizures, and have bad dreams. His groundbreaking work made some of the most critical steps forward in the field of hypnosis possible. Through his works, Avicenna showed that hypnosis was not just a mysterious or supernatural event but a natural therapeutic method that could improve people's health and well-being.

"In every studied case of recovery from hopeless and untreatable disease, there has been this major shift in consciousness so that the attractor patterns that resulted in the pathologic process no longer dominated."

– Dr. David Hawkins

A lot has changed about hypnotism over the years, from its start as a religious or mystical practice to its present use as supportive therapy. It is no longer used for regular medical treatments but is often considered a complementary service. Because of this shift in thinking, hypnotherapy is now generally seen as an excellent way to help people deal with the many problems they face in modern life.

Numerous medical conditions have been successfully treated with hypnosis. It has worked very well for people who want to stop smoking, lose weight, have trouble sleeping, deal with worry, low self-esteem, and several phobias. Still, how well the treatment works depends on the client's attitude—how serious they are about dealing with the problem they came for help with—and how open they are to hypnosis.

A common mistake about hypnosis is that it puts the person in a deep trance state where they don't know what's going on around them. Due to this misconception, many people think they can't be hypnotized and have never been in a trance. It is important to note that light trance, deep trance, and higher levels of hypnosis are all different and can be used in various ways in hypnotherapy.

Different levels of hypnosis have various effects on people. For instance, someone in a light trance can be extremely relaxed and still accept the suggestion to change a habit. The impact of a medium trance is forgetfulness, pain relief, changes in perceptions of events, and prior beliefs. Deep trance can facilitate unconscious memories that need reprocessing to benefit a new perspective, allowing forgiveness and mental healing.

Hypnotherapists typically belong to organizations that train, test, and certify hypnotists. Many are also part of regulatory groups or councils. Hypnosis has become a well-respected treatment option. It has been shown to help a wide range of issues, so anyone who wants to improve their mental and emotional health can benefit greatly.

Complementary Medical Hypnotism

People are becoming increasingly aware of the value of hypnosis as we work to overcome the stigma of Hollywood movies and the stage theatrics of hypnosis. Hypnotism is a serious science that studies and works with the subconscious mind and offers an ever more significant body of evidence for making a difference in people's lives with the many therapies offered. Sometimes, people consider hypnosis as a last resort. Still, in many cases, it should be given equal consideration in every system of medicine to work in conjunction with prescribed treatments. Hypnosis is versatile because of the many benefits it produces. Including being the best source for healing and wholeness, Hypnosis is a great support system for doctors and other practitioners as it can provide the mental stamina and the belief we need for constructive change and healing.

The root word of healing is hale, or to make whole. Healing may or may not apply to what is commonly labeled physical health. The purpose of healing is not just to return a body or mind to what society considers normal. Soul/mind/body healing should be to become a better, more self-aware individual on every level. Healing should be something that facilitates one to move towards wholeness. It is impossible to separate what is mental from the physical or spiritual from the cognitive. Most problems, unless they're at the cellular level, are spiritual, then mental, then physical, and yet our language does not offer concepts to understand these connections.

Medical hypnosis, also called hypnotherapy, is a science that studies and uses methods that tap into the subconscious mind to help people heal and improve. Doctors and other professionals can use this multipurpose tool and recommend treatments to help people change for the better. Hypnosis is not just a last resort; it works well with all medical systems.

Medical hypnosis tries to make a person whole instead of just bringing their mental or physical state back to what is expected by society. All stages of sickness are seen as out of balance, and healing means getting better and more self-aware. With complementary medical hypnosis, all three ways of healing can be made better. Getting in touch with the "doctor within" and the inner mind helps with healing and balance. This can help you break out of bad habits and choices. People can also improve their health and well-being by using hypnosis to become more spiritually aware, artistic, and able to make their dreams come true.

Here are some good things about Medical Hypnosis:

- Freedom and calmness

- Using positive self-talk to deal with stress

- Putting old designs and tools to use

- Higher levels of consciousness and awareness

- Taking care of the "doctor within."

Hypnosis is emphasized in the subconscious mind, as it plays an essential role in our behaviors. Hypnotists study the effects of the subconscious mind in our daily lives and how it plays a role in illnesses, disease, and getting well. It is an art/science since there is artistic value in utilizing suggestion therapy, imagery, and ritual. Hypnotists also do research and gather evidence regarding the subconscious mind so it can address and reframe old patterns. We must understand that the unconscious mind controls all functions of growth and balance in our body, including all dysfunction and imbalance in our bodies and social lives. With regression work and other therapy tools, getting to an issue is quick compared to many therapies focusing on cognitive thinking. Hypnosis also works by suggestion to de-emphasize old, outdated experiences, still creating trauma or re-action patterns that cause undesirable choices.

Hypnosis uses many variations of Integrative and Transpersonal Medicine. Gaining spiritual awareness once a person has entered a state of hypnosis has a powerful effect on the conscious mind, another source of disease. Regression therapy, both age and past life, to reframe old experiences triggering undesirable response patterns in our current lives is just one example. Experiencing a spiritual connection firsthand is a natural function of the higher mind once completely relaxed from everyday conscious or analytical thought. Hypnosis focuses on the most potent aspects of the human mind, imagination, and visualization, which directly correlate to manifesting reality.

One of the most recognized uses is the work done by Dr. O. Carl Simonton at the Simonton Cancer Center, where visualization is one of the primary tools used to help and heal tens of thousands of patients and as an adjunctive method of cancer treatment based on the premise that the mind and emotions can stimulate the body's immune system to fight cancer cells.

Hypnosis is then the tool for communicating with this master part of ourselves. A Hypnotist is a guide who facilitates our natural ability to access this communication. All three of these healing systems are a soul/mind/ body concept of healing, where we can become part of the process, the essential part of bringing our lives back into balance and optimum health. These systems and concepts teach us that we are the reason for imbalance and balance. Being in control of our health and wellness should be the strongest motivator of all healing efforts.

Hypnosis and Reimprinting

Hypnosis and reimprinting are two types of hypnotherapies that can help people overcome bad memories by offering the subconscious mind a better choice. The goal is to help clients let go of any emotions connected to the memory so they can move on in a better and more functional way. This approach could benefit clients with negative emotions, self-doubt, or limiting beliefs from past events.

"Conscious and unconscious thought, emotions, and intents create reality. When they are aligned, we become the reality that we prefer, if we are following our excitement, representing the natural flow of the universe."

– Lyssa Royal Holt, Mystic.

The reimprinting process has three main parts. The first step is to find the memory chain that is giving you trouble. In this step, we work with the subject to determine which memory or memories are causing the issue. A client may have test anxiety because they were made fun of for being too nervous in the past. The hypnotherapist can help the client change their memory once they have found it.

"It's never what happens to a person that remains in the memory banks and has the lasting effect, but what that person thinks, feels, decides and remembers about the event."

– William J Baldwin, Spirit Releasement

The second step in reimprinting is "fixing the inner child." To help the client's younger self (the "child") solve the problem, you need to give them valuable tools. By providing unconditional love, mature knowledge as the adult self, confidence that you'll always be with them, and always be truthful, the inner child gains the confidence to re-experience an event alongside the adult self, and new support and security of the experience is created. All subsequent events associated with the experience can now be experienced confidently up to the present moment and beyond. Typically, in a progression experience, emotion is no longer valid.

Fixing the other actors in a "memory" is about reimprinting. This means helping the person change their thoughts about the people connected to the memory. If a client's older sibling picked on them, a hypnotherapist could help them see their sibling not as a monster but as a flawed person who was misbehaving because they were jealous or felt unsafe themselves. This can help the client let go of negative feelings like anger or resentment, which can help them see the situation more clearly and with more compassion.

"Holding on to anger is like grasping a hot coal with the intent of throwing it at someone else; you are the one who gets burned."

– Buddha

The reimprinting method could help clients with many things, including getting over negative self-talk or self-doubt, anger at parents or siblings, bullying or taunting, painful experiences, and more. With this method, the client is assisted in developing a new story to help them deal with their problems healthily and powerfully. By reimprinting the memory, the person can return to their life with more hope and confidence.

"Uncovering memory and meaning are never over until life is over."

– Daniel J. Siegel, Mindsight

One of the most important things to remember when reimprinting is choosing memories that make you feel good over those that make you feel bad. The goal is to help the client create a good memory that makes them feel strong and boosts their self-esteem instead of a bad memory that brings them down. Getting the client's permission before reimprinting is vital because memories are private and personal. Remember that how you see and respond to a memory may differ from how someone else sees it. This is because everyone sees memories differently. Reimprinting aims to get around these filters and give the memory a new, better meaning.

"Spiritual process is about distancing yourself from your memory. Your memory should be a platform you stand upon to reach out for something higher, not a trap you sink into."

– Sadhguru

Although dealing with memories is a requirement for both reimprinting and regression, their methods vary. Reimprinting involves taking care of the client's younger self and changing how the client sees the other people in the memory simultaneously. When people undergo regression, they often return to a memory and work with their younger selves. Reimprinting offers a more comprehensive approach that can help clients with a broader range of issues, even though regression is helpful for healing from traumatic events.

Reimprinting and hypnosis are good ways to help people overcome painful memories and become happier and more independent. By replacing negative memories with positive ones, clients can break free from the chains of their past. This helps with self-esteem, self-worth, and believing in themselves to have their chosen lives.

Forgiveness

"Forgiveness is not an occasional act. It is a permanent attitude."

– Martin Luther King, Jr.

The healing process must include forgiveness, and hypnosis can significantly aid. Instead of ignoring or rationalizing wrongdoing, true forgiveness is letting go of the guilt and shame of dealing with painful memories. Harboring negative emotions like wrath, resentment, and bitterness can cause physical and mental harm. Forgiveness needs courage, strength, and the ability to let go.

"The weak can never forgive. Forgiveness is the attribute of the strong."

– Mahatma Gandhi

Through hypnosis, the subconscious mind can access unresolved emotions and memories. In a secure and controlled setting, hypnosis allows a person to relive the traumatic incident, processing and releasing the emotions linked to it. This might result in a more complete comprehension of the circumstances and a change in viewpoint, opening the door to forgiveness.

"Forgiveness means: You will no longer feel angry, but you might feel sadness, pity, or compassion towards the offender."

– Calvin Bayan, Hypnotherapist

As a result, the healing process might start. One way hypnosis can aid in this process is by allowing people to let go of the emotions tied to traumatic experiences in the past. Many therapists understand that ninety-five percent of an individual's conflicts occur before age seven.

The ability to recast one's viewpoint on past events, looking back as a wiser, more mature person, helps the inner child understand an event from a different perspective. This makes understanding and letting go of the emotion supporting any anger or belief easier. When one is angry, it must find physical manifestation outwardly or inwardly, but it must find expression, a view held by many.

The conscious mind must remember to comprehend the issue better and perceive things from a new perspective. Thus, one can conclude that the perpetrators' acts were frequently motivated by their lack of knowledge, terror, or suffering rather than malicious intent. People might forgive and move past their anger and resentment if they change their perspective.

"Forgiveness is correcting the misperception that someone intentionally meant to harm you."

- Jerry Jampolsky

Hypnosis can facilitate the practice of self-compassion and understanding, helping individuals learn to forgive themselves and others. Pent-up animosity and resentment can lead to persistent negative emotions of shame, remorse, and self-blame. People can let go of these negative emotions through hypnosis and cultivate a more empathetic and understanding outlook. Instead of focusing on the wrongdoer, forgiveness focuses on the victim's ability to recover and move on, more accessible, wiser, and joyful.

"Forgiveness is for you, not the offender; for your capacity to heal your life."

— Dr. Jack Kornfield

I cannot leave this subject without one of my most favored traditions of healing and making things right: the Native Hawaiian practice of Ho'oponopono. This practice utilizes the understanding of connectedness to all people and the Universe. The prayer is simple yet powerful. It captures a slight essence of the Ho'oponopono practice and can guide us through our reconciliation process when needed.

"I'm sorry.

Please forgive me.

Thank you.

I love you."

"We forgave and were forgiven, thrashing out every grudge, peeve, or sentiment among us. In this way, we become a very closely bound family unit."

– Mary Kawena Pukui

Healing and Recovery

If you want to improve, being kind and loving to yourself is most important. Forgiving others is an essential part of improving, and when we do that, we also forgive ourselves, and the bad feelings that came from the problem go away. First, we must let go of the heavy feelings holding us back.

If you want to heal the body, you must first heal the mind.

– Plato

All illnesses have physical, mental, and spiritual parts. If you want to reach the highest level of healing, all three levels must be dealt with simultaneously and given equal weight. According to this holistic viewpoint, our physical health, emotional state, and spiritual state are all dependent on one another for our well-being. How we heal and how long it lasts depends on how we see and deal with these interconnected factors.

"The body is the reflection of the spirit in its physical expression, and its problems are the dramatization of the struggles of the spirit that gives it life."

– Dr. David Hawkins

The mending process has five essential steps. First, we need to stop battling the physical signs of our illness. To do this, we must accept and welcome our present state. Second, we shouldn't name or label the sickness because that can give it a sense of self and make us think even worse things about it. Third, we shouldn't worry about saying anything. We should be in the present moment and completely immersed in our thoughts and bodily experiences. As the fourth step, we need to let go of any negative ways of thought that are linked to illness. Finally, we need to choose the Love energy. The kind of love that has no limits is quick to forgive and is marked by understanding and kindness.

"Your attitude toward your symptoms and you are critical during this healing. Your symptoms or problem is your friend. Your symptom is a signal that a creative change is needed in your life."

– Ernest Lawrence Rossi, Psychobiology of Mind-Body Healing

We should let go of any negative labels or meanings given to us or attached to our illness. We remind ourselves that we oversee our thoughts and feelings. We're in an age where everything seemingly wrong with us has a label. We give labels the power instead of ourselves. Healing is facilitated by focusing on proper functioning while visualizing an area of imbalance as healed and operating normally.

"As with determining the cause of disease, the definition, diagnosis, and classification of medical problems are highly subjective and vary from time to time and country to country. In France, for example, people with migraine headaches are likely to be diagnosed as having a liver disorder, in the United States with a vascular disorder, and in England with a gastrointestinal level."

– Lynn Payer, Medicine and Culture

This makes the "naming ceremony" a ritual in the truest sense. Symptoms are subjectively labeled into a subjective diagnosis with cultural validity. Thus, the potential for cure or control is more prescribed, and the anxiety of the patient and family must buy into treatment. You must go deeper into self-evaluation and take responsibility equally on a transpersonal approach. Healing is a combined effort of all healing methods. Each offers tools that can be used and are self-empowering.

"...for every condition in our lives, there's a "need for it." The symptom is only an outer effect. We must go within to dissolve the mental cause. This is why willpower and discipline don't work. You're only battling the outer effect. It's like cutting the weed instead of getting the root out. We must work on the "willingness to release the need" that created the condition. When the need is gone, the outer effect must die."

– Louise Hay, "Heal Your Body."

During hypnosis, we can help clients become aware of negative thoughts that hold them back and then work to replace them with more potent, more positive thoughts. Neuroscience tells us that every thought, every reverberation you create on the level of the mind, changes the chemistry in your body. By getting to know their clients' minds and helping them understand their thoughts, feelings, and actions, hypnotherapists can help their clients change the verbiage of how they think about their lives and illnesses.

The link between the mind, body, and spirit is at the heart of hypnosis and hypnotic work. By working with the subconscious mind, hypnotherapists help people heal and get back on their feet in many ways. An all-inclusive approach to healing recognizes how the physical, mental, and spiritual parts all work together, as hypnosis treats the whole person, not just the signs or labels of a specific illness. Hypnotherapists can help their clients heal and get better faster and better if they understand and deal with this dependency.

"A major study of four hundred spontaneous remissions of cancer, interpreted by Elmer & Alyce Green of the Menninger Clinic, found that all the patients had only one thing in common- every person had changed their attitudes before the remission occurred, finding some way to become hopeful, courageous, and positive."

– Deepak Chopra, Quantum Healing

Healing and Transforming Your Life

One's transformation process consists of four main elements if meaningful change is to occur. The first strategy is finding the underlying ideas, behaviors, and beliefs behind a person's concerns and issues. This means returning to the causative events or episodes that shaped these patterns—which can arise in this life, the womb, or even past lifetimes. The person can better understand the underlying dynamics at play by recognizing the primary mental root of these issues.

The second strategy emphasizes releasing the buried emotions and residue the ego has accumulated in the complexes created in response to past traumas. This is crucial since it lets the person discharge their emotional baggage. By releasing these feelings, the person can reject problematic behaviors and ideas.

Another strategy is spiritual harmony and bringing divine presence back into places where past tragedies occurred. This means calling on the client's higher self to aid in a healing process. This can be significant since it enables the person to reevaluate their prior events and grow in better knowledge of themselves and their path.

A crucial strategy also involves experiencing past incarnations. Once done, a person may connect with the Light or Soul self, where advice from a higher level of consciousness can describe how the incarnation brought a new perspective that supported an evolutionary purpose.

This can be a valuable approach to combining the knowledge and insights gained from past events and giving the person's path closure and completeness. Moreover, the person could regress to the planning stage before conception, bringing the energy and condition of that time forward to events in the womb or the present life. This can enable one to find more profound trends and themes in one's personal life.

The entire process causes the person to see their life and themselves differently. Their behaviors and actions have changed due to shifting attraction fields and signature beliefs, altering relationships, interests, and general life experiences. One can lead a more honest and contented life without reflecting on relationship experiences or reactionary patterns. The fact that modifications are a natural result of the transformation process makes one the greater since no follow-up work or maintenance is necessary.

The following is a summary of principles presented by Eric Kandel, 2000 Nobel Prize in Physiology:

Memories are not set in stone, so we can reinterpret and rework our earlier events to produce changes in the present and the future. Conscious meditation on memories and experiences helps us rewire our brains to create fresh, more empowering stories.

Emotion underlies memory formation. This view holds that emotional management can change memory storage and recall mechanisms. By deliberately practicing emotional control and reinterpreting negative emotions, we can change our memory of events.

Relationships are the foundation for vital growth. This concept stresses the need for good relationships to advance change and development. Through positive relationships and participation in therapeutic or coaching contacts, we can use social support to drive personal growth.

Nature and natural win. This theory holds that our surroundings and experiences help to define our brains and thoughts. We may change our brains to help good transformation by deliberately creating a conducive environment and engaging in activities to promote development.

Experiences transform the central nervous system. This hypothesis holds that our brains are flexible and can react to our experiences. Deliberately seeking novel experiences and practicing new skills might rewire our brains to support development and progress.

Imagining and doing are the same in brain functionality. This hypothesis implies that visualizing and mental imagery can be valuable tools for learning new abilities and changing our lives, as imagining and doing have equal brain functionality. We can boost our learning and development through deliberate imagery and mental rehearsal.

"We don't always know how or what our brain is thinking. Unconscious processes significantly influence our thoughts, actions, and feelings. The brain may process nonverbal and unconscious information, and information handled unconsciously can still influence therapeutic and other relationships. Reacting to unconscious perceptions without consciously understanding their action is possible."

– Eric Kandel, 2000 Nobel Prize in Physiology

We only sometimes know how or what our brain is thinking. This suggests that our unconscious mind significantly shapes our ideas, emotions, and behavior. Through mindfulness and self-reflection on purpose, we can become more aware of our unconscious tendencies and choose deliberately to change them.

These ideas suggest that with the intentional practice of self-reflection, emotional control, visualization, and skill development, we can use our brains to propel favorable change and growth. We might rewire our brains to support our goals and aspirations by setting a conducive atmosphere, building good connections, and practicing deliberate activities.

Chapter 10:
Self-Hypnosis And Auto Suggrstion

"Excellence is never an accident. It is always the result of high intention, sincere effort, and intelligent execution; it represents the wise choice of many alternatives - choice, not chance, determines your destiny."

—Aristotle

Self-hypnosis is not just a tool but a powerful ally in our journey towards self-control and healing. It helps us focus our minds and make the most of our skills. More importantly, it empowers us to take charge of our well-being. Hypnotherapists create a unique way to help their clients change by using their beliefs and the client's own words. The client's words become the language used to transform undesirable issues powerfully.

The body and mind are intricately connected. Every physical ailment has an emotional root, and every emotional disturbance manifests physically. The goal of any healing method is to resolve these burdensome energies or experiences. This holistic approach allows individuals to live more fully in the present and in harmony with themselves and their lives.

While conscious awareness of our behaviors is beneficial, it's equally crucial to recognize that old emotional patterns persist even after comprehending the reasons behind each issue. To take full responsibility for our experiences, we must grasp the beliefs that underpin our issues. Changing these beliefs can lead to profound mental and physical transformations.

We must also understand that some basic laws and principles govern all life. We are not living just one life; we are the sum of all life experiences. The law of attraction works simultaneously at all levels of existence: past, present, future, and multiple dimensions. When there appears to be a dysfunction, what we experience in the world around us and what we experience mentally/emotionally within us reflects painful experiences and beliefs that have not been fully processed or brought to understanding. Thus, we create and attract events to teach us where our beliefs are in error. We all measure ourselves against a hidden standard of perfection, the perfection of being a spark of God-consciousness. "Ye are all Gods."

"The ego builds up emotional residues of anger, resentment, guilt, remorse, disgust, fear, feelings of lack and scarcity, obligation or debt when it does not meet its expectations or live up to its standards."

– William Baldwin, Ph.D., Spirit Releasement Therapy

True healing in the present moment involves resolving the unfinished business of the past, which continues to influence a person in the present moment. Past events' residual mental, emotional, physical, and spiritual energy contaminates the present experience.

Emotional problems often manifest as physical illnesses, and the same is true for the other way around. Although you must be aware of your actions, old emotional habits, and beliefs may not disappear even after you understand what's causing them.

For us to heal, all healing modalities, including self-help and spiritual tools, must be used together. Healing involves pursuing knowledge and wholeness, which goes beyond physical well-being. It combines mental, physical, and spiritual parts to become our Universal selves.

"Healing in the present moment involves resolving the unfinished business of the past, which continues to influence a person in the present moment. Past events' residual mental, emotional, physical, and spiritual energy contaminates the present experience. Resolving the removal of burdensome energies is the goal of any healing approach. Then a person can live more fully in the present and fulfill more completely the details of the life plan..."

– William J Baldwin, Ph.D.

There are many important things to consider when it comes to healing. Everyone heals differently, and what works for one person might not work for another. The reasons why people get sick and have disorders are complicated and vary from person to person. Cultural views often affect how we understand the relationship between causes and effects. Symptoms may also show up in different ways, such as physically, spiritually, or socially, and treatments should be adapted to these ways.

Imagery is highly effective when manifested in a focused state. The mind can enlist imagery to assist a person in symbolically manifesting the imagined conditions. For instance, if a person with cancer sees their cells as diseased and ill, they may be instructed to imagine them transformed into healthy, vibrant cells through hypnosis. When using visualization to reach goals or make changes, we must focus on the desired positive outcome.

"Simply put, everybody's behavior makes sense to them, or they wouldn't do it. This means the crucial task of understanding someone else involves figuring out their perspective. It's not judgment. It's about radical empathy...the important thing to remember is that there are many different ways of interpreting any given situation, even one as seemingly straightforward as twenty charging horses."

– Dr. Ellen Langer, Social Psychologist at Harvard

In his book "Raising Your Children with Hypnosis" Don Mottin, Vice-President of the National Guild of Hypnotists, wrote of a study about a test where groups of students were to throw balls through a basketball hoop from the free throw line. One group was told to do nothing in preparation, while another group was told to practice every day for a specified time. A third group was told to "imagine" throwing the ball through the hoop daily for a specified time. When the groups were physically tested to determine which group would get the most balls through the hoop, guess who won...the third group won! When we are determined to do anything, we first imagine and visualize our success. Can this same process be used to heal our lives?

When someone is fully focused and exhibits a concentration of mental effort, ideas that reflect their desires are more consequential to the mind. Additionally, hypnosis is often utilized in a manner that allows deep self-exploration and discovery of unconscious intentions, motivations, events, and experiences that result in symptoms undesirable to a person. As we know, meditation and hypnosis circumvent our conscious thought processes, allowing us to gain a better insight into the problem at hand. By doing this, real change can occur.

"Each patient carries their own doctor inside. When we let the doctor that lives inside each patient do their job, they are at their best."

– Albert Schweitzer

This quote stresses the importance of people taking an active role in rehabilitation instead of depending solely on outside sources. If we accept that each person has unique needs and situations, we can work toward a more complete and adequate healing process.

Self-Hypnosis and Change

"Change will not come if we wait for another person or another time. We are the ones we've been waiting for. We are the change that we seek."

– Barack Obama

"Change" goes against our instinct for consistency and can be challenging. Homeostasis is the most potent force in human behavior. It is the enemy of change, as humans have an innate drive to stay the same, even in abusive situations. The "known" is preferable to change since consistency produces security.

In biology, homeostasis is the state of steady internal physical and chemical conditions maintained by living systems. This optimal functioning condition for the organism includes many variables, such as body temperature and fluid balance, that must be kept within certain proper functions to survive. We need steady incremental change, where the message is delivered to the subconscious mind. This can happen by reviewing how the personality was developed and the events experienced. We must correct misbeliefs that we are broken!

Recipe for Success

Understand that the subconscious mind is a goal machine. It consistently achieves what it's programmed to achieve and doesn't distinguish between good and bad. The subconscious needs daily reinforcement when changing habits and routines, as we need to resist homeostasis. We must learn to communicate with the subconscious through its language, which is symbolic language, imagination, daydreams, and bodily function and senses. Handwriting analysis is a form of symbolic language that comes directly from the subconscious and defines how you respond at that moment. You only need to see the result and work towards it daily. And don't forget the fundamental golden rule of the subconscious mind: it does not process negatives. Negatives are only reverted to positive regardless of implication because the subconscious is a positive imagining unit for the future. "I don't want to be sick" is processed as "I want to be sick." When you say that, think of how the body reacts to the thought—an experience of stress relaying "threat" to the subconscious.

"Either plan or take action to move you in the direction you want to go, or you try to cope with the thoughts, feelings, and experiences that threaten to overwhelm you."

- Richard Bandler, Guide to Transformation

We don't get what we deserve; we get what we ask for. So, see yourself moving from one successful event to the next successful event. It's also imperative to place a worth or value on the achievement. Remember everything that happens to you; your subconscious made it happen. Once you reach your goal – rewrite your contract, commitment, and a new goal.

There are many benefits to self-hypnosis, which can be broken down into four main groups: mental and emotional, physical, spiritual-metaphysical, and practical. Researchers have shown that self-hypnosis can help lower stress and worry by putting the mind and body into a deep state of relaxation. This has benefits for both the mind and the emotions. This can also lead to better attention, concentration, and cognitive abilities. People who practice self-hypnosis regularly may also notice a significant change in their self-confidence and self-esteem, making them feel more powerful and in charge of their lives.

"Whatever a person believes is real, or takes for granted as being real, is real in its consequences."

– W.I. Thomas, Clinical Sociologist

In addition, self-hypnosis can be very helpful for emotional recovery because it creates a safe and supportive space for people to face and heal emotional scars and past traumas. By getting into the subconscious mind, self-hypnosis can help people change negative thought patterns and behaviors, leading to a more decisive positive attitude.

"Changed behavior can only come from changing belief systems and from the way we generalize our experience."

– Richard Bandler, Guide to Transformation

Self-hypnosis can also be very helpful for changing bad habits and behaviors, like stopping smoking or losing weight, by reprogramming the subconscious mind to form healthier and more positive habits. Extensive research has shown that self-hypnosis is an excellent way to deal with and lessen chronic pain or emotional stress. Inducing a deep state of relaxation through self-hypnosis can help reduce inflammation and speed up healing, which is good for your general health and well-being. Self-hypnosis can help with trouble sleeping, which is essential for your health and well-being. It also allows the immune system to lower stress and promote relaxation. This frees up the immune system to fight off infections and diseases. It is possible to lower your blood pressure and lower your risk of heart disease and other heart problems by practicing self-hypnosis regularly. Relaxation reduces anxiety and depression, both of which can negatively impact the immune system. Improved mental health through relaxation contributes to overall well-being and a more resilient immune response.

"Every thought affects every part of the body...our immune responses begin in the brain."

– Dr. Ellen Langer

Self-hypnosis can help you feel more peaceful and calmer on the inside, which is good for your general health. It also has spiritual and metaphysical benefits. Letting people reach their subconscious and calm their minds can help them develop their intuition and gain deeper spiritual insights. This can make people feel more connected to their inner selves and the world. Individuals can feel more centered and grounded when they use self-hypnosis. This can help them find a more profound sense of purpose and direction by linking with their spiritual guardians or higher self.

"Until a new and better habit is securely rooted, no exceptions must be allowed. You cannot even once revert to the old bad habit."

– William James, Psychologist

One of the best things about self-hypnosis is how easy it is to use. You can do it in very little time, which makes it perfect for people who are always on the go. Also, self-hypnosis is an inexpensive way to improve your mental and physical health. The most important thing about self-hypnosis is that it lets people take charge of their own emotional and physical health. People can live a more meaningful and satisfying life by taking an active role in their healing and development, which can boost their confidence and self-assurance.

Step-by-Step Guide to Self-Hypnosis

Here are step-by-step directions for how to do self-hypnosis.

Step 1: FIND A COMFORTABLE POSITION

Wear clothes to feel relaxed. A comfortable, easy chair works best.

Step 2: FIND THE PEACEFUL PLACE

Pick out a quiet room, put your phone on silent, and lie down in a way that supports your back.

Step 3: CLEARLY STATE YOUR GOAL

Before you exercise, have a clear goal, such as boosting your confidence, getting better sleep, or stopping a bad habit.

Step 4: FOCUS YOUR ATTENTION ON ONE THING

Find a simple focus point in your line of sight, like a candle flame or a colored thumbtack on the wall. Focus your mind on this spot to help you concentrate. You can also look up slightly to put a little tension on your eye lids.

Step 5: BREATHE SLOWLY AND DEEPLY

Keep your eyes on the central point as you slowly breathe in through your nose and out through your mouth. Imagine that each time you breathe, your eyes get heavier until they are too heavy to keep open.

Step 6: STAY CALM AND RELAXED

While keeping your eyelids closed, keep breathing slowly and pay attention to your breath to keep your mind from moving. Should your thoughts stray, gently bring your attention back to your breath. If you feel tension, picture the strain leaving your body with each exhalation.

Step 7: PICTURE IT

Use all your senses to develop a calm, happy place. For example, picture yourself on a quiet beach surrounded by peaceful clouds. Make sure that your mental picture is as clear and thorough as possible.

Step 8: INTENSIFY YOUR RELAXATION

As you focus on your thoughts, picture your body getting heavy, like you are about to fall asleep. Should it help, picture yourself slowly sinking into the couch or chair.

Step 9: FEEL CALM AND LET YOUR ENERGY DRAIN AWAY

To strengthen your peace, say a phrase to yourself, for example, "I am at peace" or "I am calm."

Step 10: MOVE ON TO YOUR GOAL

When you are completely calm, use your imagination to focus on your goal. Make sure that your image is as clear and vivid as possible. For example, if you want to sleep better, picture yourself in a soft, cozy bed with soft blankets, breathing deeply in the cool darkness while listening to the soft hum of the fan.

Step 11: INTENSIFY YOUR GOAL AND IMAGE

As you picture yourself reaching your goal, repeat affirmations to yourself repeatedly, for example, "I am speaking with confidence" or "I am sleeping peacefully through the night." Be kind to yourself and encourage yourself as you repeat these affirmations.

Step 12: EASING OUT OF TRANCE

Imagine that each breath takes energy from the air around you and sends it flowing through your body. Your limbs feel lighter with each breath until they return to their awakened state.

Step 13: AWAKEN REFRESHED READY FOR A FANTASTIC DAY

As you count down from 10, tell yourself, "When I reach one, I will awaken feeling refreshed, alert, and full of energy." This will help you gradually emerge from the unconscious and reach full awareness.

Rules and Power of the Subconscious Mind

The conscious mind evaluates and compares each new idea with previously accepted ideas and then sends it to the subconscious. The conscious mind can reason and decide your actions. Will-power cannot override what has been programmed as a valid belief or response. It will raise a barrier between the subconscious and a new suggestion, preventing its penetration until it is reinforced. That's why habits cannot be broken by the conscious mind alone. The subconscious needs proof that a change has occurred through the body's reactions before it becomes supportive of a new conscious activity or habit.

"The subconscious will attempt to complete whatever is the strongest task in your mind."

– Terence Watts, British Hypnotherapist

Our decisions are always based on the strength of our desires. Subconscious responses outweigh conscious desires. Unless the subconscious is changed, habits of thinking dominate one's actions. The subconscious does not discriminate between helpful and detrimental ideas. For example, hearing a negative statement several times as a young child, "You never do anything right," leads to a subconscious memory that reinforces that belief as an adult. Since the subconscious mind does not have a critical ability, it accepts as absolute truth any idea allowed in. This can become a child's belief and consequent behavior. When a suggestion is offered, the subconscious mind accepts only what the conscious mind believes.

Suppose the conscious mind changes an opinion after it's entrenched. In that case, the subconscious will not change unless we bypass an old response with a new response, in which the feelings,

194

body, and actions respond differently. With a continued new reaction over a few weeks, the subconscious will recognize it and become supportive. Also, when challenged with a competing positive response and negative memory, the subconscious will always choose a positive response versus a negative one. Later in life, the never-do-it-right can be changed, visualizing the successes in life and re-experiencing the feelings and emotions connected to the achievements. Once that is reinforced daily through affirming self-talk and action, it becomes an entrenched habit of thinking and belief. Self-hypnosis, visualization of a new action, and Neurolinguistic Programming can speed up this process.

Convincing the Subconscious Mind

Repetition is the key to results. I use the example of watching a commercial. If you see a commercial one time, chances are you will scan all the same products. But! If you see that same commercial a thousand times, you will likely choose that product because of the color, labeling, logo, packaging, and other distinguishing characteristics. The reasoning is simple: since watching a commercial, your conscious mind is less active, and having seen the commercial before, there's no critical analysis needed. The commercial sinks into the subconscious mind, becoming more actively alert as the commercial no longer has the conscious mind's attention. Advertisers use this knowledge. Why spend millions of dollars advertising for you to stand in front of their product together with like products, consciously deciding which product to buy? They would prefer to use the speed of the subconscious to choose their product because it is recognizable automatically, and your choice is made very quickly without forethought.

Identification with a group or parent is another automatic response. This is your typical programming and conditioning. When your mother says, "You're just like your father," or you have your father's "Irish temper," this becomes ingrained for life or whenever you choose to reprogram to no longer act in such a way.

How about authority figures you admire? Their ideas, actions, dress, and all other things about them are copied into your life. The subconscious mind uses mimicry to learn at a very early age. President Kennedy was a hero of mine, and I spoke like him and presented his inaugural address speech at a school talent contest. The famous quote, "Ask not what your country can do for you, but what you can do for your country," resonates in my mind sixty years later.

Intense emotions open a corridor directly to the subconscious mind, where the emotion can become a threat. Especially since the subconscious mind always asks, "Am I safe?" repeatedly throughout the day with every bodily reaction. Anxieties and stress reactions are responded to as a threat. For example, you show up at work five minutes late. Your conscious mind runs the tape of possible trouble, such as if I will be fired, how I will pay my bills, the mortgage, and all sorts of drama, even though you think it's not a problem. Your brain is wired like your Neanderthal brothers or sisters; if you were late, you could be eaten.

Whether you use self-hypnosis or a hypnotist, you can evaluate an issue and use suggestions to reframe the subconscious response and new actions. Suggestions must be tailored to your specific challenge. With self-hypnosis, you can structure a suggestion in your own words, which is more potent than another's words. But it does take practice. Statements do not work since saying "I want to quit smoking" is not bypassing the conscious mind, so the subconscious may or may not take you seriously. Even with a smoking cessation session, reinforcement is still needed until enough time has passed with the desired reaction.

"Until a new and better habit is securely rooted, no exceptions must be allowed. You cannot even once revert to the old bad habit."

– William James, Psychologist

Principles of Structuring a Suggestion

1. MOTIVATING DESIRE MUST BE STRONG

   a. Before you write your suggestion, choose a reason or several reasons why you want your suggestion carried out. This must be a counter-emotional motivator to replace the behavior pattern you intend to eliminate.

   b. Start your suggestion with your motivating desire.

   i. *"I strongly desire an attractive, slim figure because I enjoy wearing a size nine dress."*

   ii. *"Because I want to feel physically fit and enjoy vibrant health."*

2. BE POSITIVE

   a. Never mention the negative idea you intend to eliminate. Repeat and emphasize the positive idea you are replacing it with.

   b. "What is expected tends to be realized." This is the law of mental expectancy.

    c. The subconscious can only respond to mental images, and the idea is to form new mental images.

    d. Self-hypnosis is positive thinking in its most practical form!

3. ALWAYS USE THE PRESENT TENSE

    a. When you read your suggestion, don't just say the words you have written. Think of them, imagine them, and see yourself acting out the suggestion.

    b. When you use your imagination, you directly contact the subconscious.

    c. Your self-image has much to do with your success or failure. If you want to be successful...visualize yourself being successful! See yourself as you want to be or visualize your goal as already accomplished, then hypnotize yourself.

4. SET A TIME LIMIT

    a. Be reasonable about how long it takes to accomplish a goal, such as a broken leg in sports.

    b. Your subconscious is a goal-striving mechanism, and once programmed toward a goal, it never stops until it achieves it!

5. SUGGEST ACTION, NOT ABILITY TO ACT

    a. Don't say, "I can dance well." Say = "I dance well, with ease and grace!"

6. BE SPECIFIC

    a. Don't suggest several things at once—alternate suggestions at different sessions, but never more than two or three at once.

7. KEEP YOUR LANGUAGE SIMPLE

    a. Talk to yourself as a bright ten-year-old.

8. EXAGGERATE AND EMOTIONALIZE

    a. The subconscious is the seat of emotions, and exciting, powerful words will influence it.

    b. Use descriptive words, i.e., wonderful, beautiful, exciting, fantastic, thrilling, joyous, gorgeous, and tremendous! With feeling!

9. USE REPETITION

    a. Repeat, enlarge upon, and repeat it in different words.

    b. Embellish it with convincing adjectives.

    c. Repeat your suggestions daily until they become entrenched in your subconscious.

    d. The brain will always send a message to act upon any suggestion unless conflicting suggestions inhibit it.

Autosuggestion

In the early 1900s, a French doctor named Émile Coué devised a way to help people called "autosuggestion." This is a type of self-induced advice in which people change their feelings, thoughts, or actions to improve their health and well-being.

Coué believed that operating below our conscious awareness was a complex assortment of ideas that can be dominant while continuously and spontaneously suggesting things to us. These ideas were valuable for supporting overall health and well-being.

"We possess within us a force of incalculable power, which, when we handle it unconsciously, is often prejudicial to us. If, on the contrary, we direct it consciously and wisely, it gives us mastery of ourselves and allows us not only to escape ... from physical and mental ills but also to live in relative happiness, whatever the conditions in which we may find ourselves."

– Emile Coue

The following basic ideas form the basis of Coué's autosuggestion:

The Dominating role of the imagination: How we imagine things dramatically affects our bodies.

Limited to physical possibility: Autosuggestion can lead to results that align with the boundaries of physical possibility.

From birth to death, we are all slaves to suggestion. Our destinies are decided by suggestion. It is a potent influence that we don't consciously realize. But we can use these hidden gems by disciplined suggestion and direct it in the way we wish; this becomes autosuggestion: we can take a conscious approach and take advantage of the hidden advice by visualizing what we want.

"Emphasis should be placed more on what we do in the present and will do in the future than on a mere understanding of why some long-past event occurred."

– Milton H. Erickson

There is proof that imagination is a dominant factor in the physical body over the experience of pain, movement, emotions, and sensations. Its effect is both moral and physical.

Essential Things to Know About Autosuggestion

The moral factor is the principle of right and wrong behavior and the decent or shameful nature of the human character. Some doctors say that our ideas and imaginations can significantly affect our health, and the moral factor may be responsible for 40–50% of recovery prospects.

"A patient who says to himself "I am getting better" vastly increases his vital forces and hastens their recovery. By gently putting our imagination on the right track, we are sure of aiding Nature, who manifests herself through the medium of the subconscious self."

– Emile Coue

The power of the imagination: By using autosuggestion, we can use our imaginations to improve our health. I purposefully avoided a root canal, eliminated a groin pain three doctors told me to live with, pulled cysts out of my wrist, and the list could go on. By using suggestion, affirmation, imagination, and personal therapy, I was able to eliminate and heal disorders.

"The instinct of self-preservation is but a manifestation of Nature."

– Emile Coue

The subconscious mind: Our inner mind is a powerful tool that we can use to improve our health and well-being. Focus all your attention on an object. Thinking stops, and the subconscious is present. Now, turn your attention to your body, breathe, and close your eyes. Scan your body. You can now shift any energy as needed. Return your attention to simply observing the breath. Relax; you're ready to do whatever you suggest. Our subconscious does not require the details. It knows much more than we can ever know about our bodies.

"That wonderful subconscious self does it. For it knows and commands every movement of our being, every contraction of our heart, the minutest of vibration of every cell in our organism."

– Emil Coue

Importance of relaxation: If you want to use autosuggestion effectively, you must avoid focusing or exerting yourself and instead relax. These actions can block the suggestion from reaching your mind. Coué advised that people say the following phrase to themselves every night before going to sleep: "Every day, in every way, I am getting better and better." Once on each fingertip. People should use this saying as general advice and can use it all their lives. People can use the power of autosuggestion to improve their health and well-being by doing it regularly, along with a visualization of being healed. This becomes a potent practice for healing.

"I declare without hesitation that whatever the illness, the practice of rational auto-suggestion will always affect an appreciation

202

improvement in the patient's condition, even if the disease itself be incurable."

– Emil Coue

Autosuggestion and The Leland Method

In New Thought philosophy, the theory of Attraction is the belief that people can bring positive or negative experiences into their lives by focusing on positive or negative thoughts. This belief is based on the idea that people and their thoughts are made from pure energy and that through the process of like energy attracting like energy, a person can improve their health, wealth, and personal relationships. The Law of Attraction is among the most popular of the Universal Laws.

"Thought is vibration, and the law of attraction brings more thought. You cannot want something you don't have and be a vibrational match. You must be what you want – and then you can have it."

– Abraham, Esther Hicks

The Leland Method, created by Charles Godfrey Leland at the turn of the century, states you can get what you want using autosuggestion. Using autosuggestion to get yourself to perform a task or have a particular thought state is part of the Leland Method. This is the very foundation of the principle of autosuggestion. Even better, if you focus on something, autosuggestion can help you realize how to develop your desires, intents, dreams, and hopes into reality.

"Sometimes all it takes is a tiny shift of perspective to see something familiar in a new light"

– Dan Brown, American author

The first step of the Leland Method, in the beginning, is to decide before bed that you will do something that requires willpower or resolution, like finishing a problematic job, facing a challenging situation, or reaching a particular mental state (like being happy). This choice should be made calmly and carefreely, without any need to be harsh or aggressive. Choose to do it, and then let your inner mind care for the rest. Diligence is essential in this process because it will give more consistent and good results if done regularly. Expecting to be outstanding immediately is unrealistic, but if you practice regularly, you will make it a habit to encourage yourself to get what you want.

As its focus, the Leland Method looks at how habits change over time. You can reach a happy state of mind by repeatedly committing to mental calmness and happiness. In the same way, removing pictures that make you feel bad will make it easier to deal with negative thoughts. You can also use this method to improve specific skills or abilities, like waking up at a particular time or remembering certain things. The key is to keep your mind on the desired result and repeatedly tell yourself the idea until it becomes second nature.

The deferred decision is another essential part of the Leland Method. A specific thought will likely come back on a particular day or time. This is because the idea is present in your subconscious mind, even when you are not consciously thinking about it. You can reach certain mental states during the day if you practice regularly. As a result, your consciousness will become more robust.

There is a difference between a firm and soft desire and a strong effort when you want to get anything that requires will or resolution. Say the goal repeatedly, calmly, and gently until you fall asleep. Focus your mind on a specific thing or outcome to start. Experiment again.

If it worked the first time, try adding more things or results. The Leland Method is based on doing things repeatedly and planning.

After bed for the night, thoroughly evaluate a want and desire. Having done this, will or declare that what you want shall pass on waking, repeating this, thinking about it, and falling asleep. Only wish for two things simultaneously, as your mind must become familiar with the process. As you feel your power strengthens with success, you may will yourself to do whatever you desire.

"If we will that a certain idea shall recur to us on the following or any other day, and if we bring the mind to bear upon it just before falling asleep, it may be forgotten when we awake, but it will recur to us when the time comes."

- Charles Godfrey Leland

Just by the same process that enables us to awake at a given hour, and simply by substituting other ideas for that of time, we can acquire the ability to bring ourselves pre-determined or desired states of mind. This is Auto-Suggestion or deferred determination, be it with or without sleep. It becomes more specific in its results with every new experiment or trial.

Overall, the significant factor is perseverance or repetition. By faith, we can remove mountains; by perseverance, we can carry them away, and the two amount to precisely the same thing. By continued practice and thought, in Autosuggestion, practicing soon finds that the conscious mind will be acting more vigorously in waking hours, no longer needing the prior-to-sleep process. When we see that our will is beginning to obey us and inspire courage and indifference where we were once timid, there is no end to the confidence and power that may ensue.

The Leland Method stresses the importance of forethought, a solid but gentle desire, and keeping at it when using autosuggestion. By following these rules, you can develop a more powerful and effective way to affect your subconscious mind and get the desired results. This method might help people get along better with others, be successful and wealthy, feel better generally, and overcome their fears and phobias. You can live a more satisfying life by using the power of autosuggestion to reach your full potential.

"You must always remember that after you have said to your subconscious, "Attend to this for me while I sleep," you must then positively dismiss the matter from your outer consciousness, just as a great executive dismisses a matter when he gives it over to a tried and trusted assistant. Until you do this, the subconscious cannot do its work properly."

— Charles Godfrey Leland

Autosuggestion Exercise

This exercise takes only a few minutes to accomplish and should be practiced at least once a day. Relax with your eyes closed. Do this exercise slowly. Repeat suggestions when indicated. Never do this while driving. This can be done silently or out loud. All it requires is your concentration. If possible, commit these suggestions to memory.

Step 1: RELAX AND PREPARE

Find a quiet and comfortable place to sit or lie down where you won't be disturbed. Close your eyes and take three deep breaths through your nose and out through your mouth. Feel your body relax and let go of any tension.

Step 2: CALM YOUR MIND

Repeat the following phrases to yourself slowly and calmly:

"I feel calm."

"I feel relaxed."

"I feel in control."

"I am calm."

"I am relaxed."

"I am in control."

"I feel safe."

"I am secure."

"I can let go."

As you say these phrases, imagine any opposing thoughts or feelings leaving your body. Feel your body relax and your mind calm.

Step 3: OPEN YOUR MIND TO POSITIVE SUGGESTIONS

Say to yourself: "My subconscious mind is now open to receiving the helpful and beneficial suggestions I'm about to give myself."

Step 4: CREATE YOUR AFFIRMATION Think about something you want to achieve or improve in your life. It could be related to your health, relationships, career, or anything important. Create a short, positive sentence that affirms your goal. For example:

"I am confident and capable in my career."

"I am worthy of love and respect."

"I am healthy and strong."

Repeat your affirmation to yourself 10 times, slowly and calmly. Imagine yourself achieving your goal and feeling happy and fulfilled.

Step 5: REINFORCE YOUR AFFIRMATION (REINFORCE YOUR AFFIRMATION (OPTIONAL)

If you want to focus on a specific physical or health-related goal, add the following phrase to your affirmation:

"For my body, I choose to [insert goal, e.g., 'be healthy and strong' or 'be free from anxiety']. My body can [insert goal], and I trust its ability to heal and thrive."

Step 6: CLOSE THE EXERCISE

Count forward from 1 to 3, and then slowly open your eyes. Take a deep breath and feel refreshed and renewed.

Remember to practice this exercise regularly, ideally twice a day, to help you relax, focus your mind, and achieve your goals.

Benefits of Hypnotic Music

Hypnotic music, characterized by repetitive rhythms, calming melodies, and ambient sounds, offers numerous benefits, particularly in therapeutic practices like hypnotherapy. Most good hypnotic music is made with binaural beats. This creates the frequency your brain uses to create the same waves commonly experienced during meditation. Binaural beats in this way are sometimes called brain wave entrainment technology. Binaural beats have been shown in studies to reduce anxiety by 26%. Helping with sleep: Certain frequencies of binaural beats activate certain brain waves, which can help the body and mind relax and sleep more deeply.

"Meditation, bliss technique, and primordial sound are the practical applications of Quantum Healing. What is happening is that the body is receiving a signal from its blueprint, not a material blueprint but the one that exists in consciousness. ...because the blueprint is invisible, it must find a way to cross over into material existence. To do that, nature employs bliss (deep meditation, hypnosis, intense focus) – using a vibration (primordial sound) that bridges mind and matter, allowing each bit of the body to be paired with a bit of intelligence."

– Deepak Chopra, Quantum Healing

Key Benefits Music:

"Real music is not for the mind or the body, but for the spirit which exists independently of each."

– Ali Akbar Khan, contemporary Indian musician

1. Relaxation and Stress Reduction

The soothing sounds and rhythms can help lower heart rate and blood pressure, promoting deep relaxation. By calming the mind, hypnotic music can alleviate stress and anxiety, providing a mental escape from daily pressures.

2. Enhanced Focus and Concentration

The repetitive nature of hypnotic music can help improve focus and concentration, making it easier to enter a meditative or trance-like state. For hypnotherapists, such music can help clients achieve the relaxed and focused state necessary for effective hypnotherapy.

3. Aid in Sleep and Insomnia Treatment

The calming effects of hypnotic music can help individuals fall asleep more quickly and enjoy more profound, restorative sleep. Regularly listening to hypnotic music can be an effective non-pharmacological treatment for insomnia.

4. Pain Management

Hypnotic music can distract from pain and discomfort, making it a valuable tool for pain management in clinical settings. It has been shown to reduce chronic pain conditions, such as fibromyalgia, by promoting relaxation and reducing muscle tension.

5. Enhanced Emotional Well-Being

Listening to calming music can enhance mood and create a sense of well-being. It can help alleviate symptoms of depression by providing an emotional outlet and promoting positive mental states.

6. Spiritual and Metaphysical Benefits

Hypnotic music can enhance spiritual practices such as meditation, visualization, and guided imagery. It can help individuals connect more deeply with their inner selves and expand their spiritual awareness.

7. Supports Behavioral Change

Hypnotic music's repetitive and calming nature can help the brain become more flexible and open to new thinking patterns. In combination with hypnotherapy, hypnotic music can aid in modifying behaviors and reinforcing positive changes.

8. Creativity and Problem-Solving

The relaxed and focused state induced by hypnotic music can enhance creative thinking and problem-solving abilities. It can help individuals tap into their intuition and subconscious mind, fostering innovative ideas and insights.

9. Physical Healing and Recovery

Hypnotic music can support physical healing and recovery by promoting relaxation and reducing stress. Its stress-reducing effects can also enhance immune function, improving overall health and well-being.

10. Customized Therapeutic Applications

Hypnotherapists can use specific types of hypnotic music to match the therapeutic goals and individual needs of their clients. Music can support guided visualization techniques, making them more vivid and compelling. By integrating hypnotic music into therapeutic practices, individuals can experience a range of physical, emotional, and spiritual benefits, enhancing overall well-being and facilitating personal growth and healing.

"Melody plays a small role. The 'sound' of the music, tonal quality, is important. (It is the component of music which is associated with the 'right hemisphere' of the brain.)"

– Robert Ornstein, "The Psychology of Consciousness"

Chapter 11:
Aligning The Mind With The Universe

"In what is seen, there must be just the seen; in what is heard, there must be just the heard; in what is sensed (taste, smell, or touch), there must be just what is sensed; in what is thought, there must be just the thought."

– Buddha

The Ego

There is much maligned about the ego in many spiritual and psychological contexts. I've heard you "must" slay the ego. That's your ego talking. The point is that everyone has an ego, including any Saint or self-aware being, including Jesus Christ. The ego serves a very positive function in our life. Without it, we couldn't survive the elements. Nor could we have any enjoyment or pleasures this world has to offer.

213

"The design function of the mind is survival of the being, or whatever the being considers itself to be."

– William Baldwin, Ph.D.

When we are born, the physical body becomes the primary identification, and the need to survive becomes the focus and the goal. Once we have developed a personality, we add the thinking mind to this need. Now, the mind is involved in the need for survival by whatever means necessary. This concern becomes our ego. The focus and function of the ego then become the evaluator of all life experiences, using any necessary thoughts and emotions to drive its need for survival.

The ego survives by seeing everything as a competition. It validates its own decisions as right, whether true or not, while making others' decisions wrong. All the while, it justifies its actions and behaviors while judging the behavior of others. Judgments, assumptions, conclusions, and decisions become the dominating way in which the ego responds. As we age, this thinking becomes the patterns and habits we build into our lives. Every natural or imagined challenge where the ego meets a perceived threat becomes part of the survival mechanism.

"The ego is...primarily engaged in defense and furthering its ambitions. Everything that interferes with it must be repressed. The repressed elements ...become the shadow."

– Jack Sanford, Jungian Analyst, Episcopal Priest

The challenge is that the ego is also the judge and jury of our life. It judges its actions against the perfection of our actual being, which is God's consciousness. Thus, the ego builds up emotional experiences of anger, resentment, guilt, remorse, disgust, fear, feelings of lack, obligation, or debt when it doesn't measure up to the potential of our actual being.

"A man's conscience is the most severe Judge when allowed to speak clearly and forcibly. Stripping aside all self-deception and hypocrisy, conscious or unconscious, it causes the soul to stand naked and bare to its spiritual gaze. And the soul, speaking as its conscience, sentences itself by its conceptions of right and wrong, and accepts its fate as merited and just."

- William Walker Atkinson, Author and American Pioneer of New Thought

So why wouldn't we want to kill off this part of our being? How could we enjoy this world if we did? Could we love, laugh, find joy and pleasure, happiness? How about responding creatively to our dreams and goals?

The ego creates a sense of self, helping us define who we are, our values, beliefs, and boundaries. The ego mind supports our personal development and self-understanding as it is in concert with the analyzing evaluating brain. This mind helps us navigate challenges and potential threats. It encourages self-preservation and the pursuit of goals that ensure survival and well-being.

The ego drives our creative desires for success. It motivates us to achieve, excel, and pursue our goals for personal growth, accomplishments, and life fulfillment. We need positive self-esteem and confidence deserving of life's good things. To enjoy the awesomeness of a magnificent world of beauty and wonder.

The ego plays a crucial role in social interactions, helping us build relationships and assess options based on our values, desires, and beliefs. It promotes autonomy and the ability to make choices that align with personal goals while supporting our unique self-expression and creativity.

The challenges posed by the ego can lead to significant personal and spiritual growth. As individuals become aware of and work through ego-driven behaviors, they can achieve higher self-awareness and spiritual development.

EGO VS. SPIRIT

One of the most transformational moments in your life is realizing there is a difference between your ego/personality and your soul/spirit. The ego mind is simply a collection of thoughts that interpret reality based on its own bias. The ego is primarily concerned with its well-being and the attraction of pleasures. A simple definition of the ego is where we derive our self-esteem, self-importance, self-worth, self-respect, self-image, and self-confidence. The ego is very self-oriented. We use the ego to project our personality, which is all housed in the critical, analytical, and conscious mind.

"Matter is the vehicle for the manifestation of soul on this plane of existence, and soul is the vehicle on a higher plane for the manifestation of spirit, and these three are a trinity synthesized by Life, which pervades all."

– H. P. Blavatsky

The soul is the fundamental truth and proposition that is the foundation for our psychical origin. It is the principle of life, feeling, intuition, and action in humans. It is regarded as a distinct entity separate from the body. Its connection is in the subconscious mind, always in the background of the conscious mind, watching and observing our existence.

"– Man is a portal through which one enters the outer world of the gods, demons, and souls into the inner world, from the greater world into the smaller world. Small and insignificant is man; one leaves him soon behind, and thus one enters once more into infinite space, into the microcosm, into the inner eternity."

– C.G. Jung

Simply put, your ego is your mask—your image of yourself, while your soul is your spirit—your essence and your true self. So, why are we dwelling so much on this mind-boggling concept of using the ego mind to define reality? This is one essential way of understanding life-based on our personal experiences and preferred perception of reality.

"You are what you think, having become what you thought."

– Buddha

The ego mind seeks to survive by validating its viewpoint and invalidating others. Judgments, conclusions, and decisions build up over lifetimes and form our beliefs about life. We rarely question our motives and thoughts when things are going as desired, especially when we get the response from others that we want to support our ego drives. If, on the other hand, you are bombarded with negative vibes, negative self-talk, and negative beliefs, the ego will defend itself by considering itself right and others wrong. This may lead us to dominate others with direct aggression or passive aggression. This can develop automatic responses without consideration of reactions or consequences.

The choice is ours. To live a choice-driven life, we must balance our lesser mind, ego/personality, and greater mind, Spirit/Soul. Using positive inner guidance for a better life, a change will start with you understanding how your lesser mind and greater mind work and can work together. Feelings will always validate thinking when acquiescing to the higher mind.

"There are three truths which are absolute and cannot be lost yet may remain silent for lack of speech: (I) The soul of man is immortal, and its future is the future of a thing whose growth and splendor have no limit. (II) The principle which gives life dwells in us, and without us, is undying and eternally beneficent, is not heard or seen or felt, but is perceived by the man who desires perception. (II) Each man is his absolute lawgiver, the dispenser of glory or gloom to himself, the decrier of his life, reward, and punishment. These truths, which are as great as life itself, are as simple as the simplest mind of man."

– The Complete Works of William Walker Atkinson

Have a Conversation with Your Gut

I introduced the solar plexus or gut brain in chapter five. Now, learning to communicate with this vital body part is essential. This complex network of neurons and microbes in our gut that talk to our brain affects our feelings, mood, and decision-making ability. We can tell if a thought is right or wrong by sending it to our gut. People often call this a "gut feeling" or intuition. We can go with an idea if it makes sense. We can turn down the idea and think about other options if it doesn't feel right.

"The past reaches into the present to program the future."

– Dr. Phil

However, the body responds to an experience, and the information is transmitted via the vagus nerve to the subconscious mind for processing. We must learn to pay attention to the body, as feelings and emotions don't lie. This can help us decipher the value of our thinking and determine where the feeling should be the final arbiter since feelings are a moment-to-moment experience. For the same reason, when we have a strong emotion, an energized feeling, we can explore our conscious mind to see if there is a threat. If not, we can put aside our feelings and explore the triggered emotion. What happened in the past might bring up emotions. This can help us learn more about our emotions and feelings, deciding on a better way to deal with them. It is always better to have a delayed response when unsure since the subconscious is much quicker than our conscious mind and does not choose positive or negative but one of protection.

"The human body is not an instrument to be used, but a realm of one's being to be experienced, explored, enriched and thereby, educated."

-Thomas Hanna, founder of Clinical Somatic Education

Anything that happens to us is by referencing everything that has already happened to us. The subconscious mind remembers every detail of every experience. These details add to our interpretation of our experiences to form our chosen reality called "patterns" of action or reaction. Once recognized by the subconscious mind, the final question becomes, "Am I safe"? If not, a response is used to ensure your safety, sometimes at great expense. Illness is an excellent example, as its ramifications alter our actions and reactions. And this occurs whether it's a real or imagined threat.

The two minds constantly communicate about everything, even the most routine affairs or a spiritual quest. The goal is to become a better person, stop sabotaging behavior, follow a sage's wisdom, or walk the talk of your personal beliefs and truths. There will always be a time when you experience conflicts between the spirit, soul, and authentic self and the fears and anxieties of the ego. In one moment, spirituality could be at the forefront, and in another moment, ego could dominate your actions and thoughts. However, your intuitive self can be felt and become more vital than your ego when making your ultimate decision.

What does that conversation sound like? It always comes through feelings. A gut-level instinct, a knowingness, a cheerful voice that triggers a noticeable positive feeling. If it feels right, accept the thoughts. If it doesn't feel right...reject the thoughts.

"Intuition is the strength of the soul...we are wired through our intuition."

– Caroline Myss, Medical Intuitive

Over time, while your true self emerges, it will challenge how you think, look at the world, and live your life. As your spiritual awareness grows more robust, your ego becomes less dominant. The ego does not have the power to act against the higher vibrations of the soul self. Just remember, negative emotions can block the vibrations of the soul self. This conflict will probably be a time of confusion and fear. Ultimately, which voice you "choose" to listen to is yours.

"When the conscious mind knows what is in the subconscious mind, you will be enlightened."

– Carl Jung

"Be Here Now"- Universe Time

"Do not worry about your life". "Who of you by worrying can add a single hour to his life?" "Why do you worry about clothes?" "Do not worry, saying, 'What shall we eat?' or "What shall we drink?' or 'What shall we wear?" "Do not worry about tomorrow"

– Matthew 6:25-34

One of the more fascinating hypnosis experiences is that clients rarely know how long they have been in hypnosis. We use this to reinforce the idea that they were in hypnosis. Many clients will say they didn't think they were in hypnosis because they were conscious. So, the hypnotist needs to dispel the idea that hypnosis is not a sleep state or even an unconscious state. This belief has come from vampire shows, television, and so on since the birth of modern hypnosis around the fifties. A client needs to believe they have been hypnotized so the conscious mind accepts the suggestion given. This is very important for hypnotic work. Typically, a client thinks they've been in hypnosis for fifteen to twenty minutes when it is anywhere from thirty to fifty minutes. There is an ah-ha moment that comes with this revelation.

"Space or time is not an object or a thing. Space is another form of our animal understanding and does not have an independent reality. We carry space and time around with us like turtles with shells. Thus, there is no absolute self-existing matrix in which physical events occur independent of life."

– Robert Lanza, Biocentric Design

This reveals that there is no time or space in the subconscious mind. Time and space are only relative to the conscious mind or observer. Einstein determined that time is relative—in other words, the rate at which time passes depends on your frame of reference. He believed that time is an illusion, that both the future and the past are unchangeable and will play out exactly how they were meant to. We all live in the third dimension and linear time, meaning the conscious mind thinks in the past, present, and future. This does present a problem since the only time is now.

"Enlightenment is understanding that there is nowhere to go, nothing to do, and nobody you have to be except exactly who you are being right now."

– Neale Donald Walsch,

The positive side of living and thinking in this dimension is that it allows us to evaluate our perspective and perception of past events. The ego or conscious mind sees reality from a personal interpretation that maintains safety. The reality we see is stored in the personal consciousness. This means that we see, evaluate, and judge by personal beliefs. In truth, time is one ten thousandths of a second, so we only experience a tiny sample of actual reality. This opens the door to misperceptions and misinterpretations of human interactions, which leads to false decisions, assumptions, and conclusions. The events must be re-experienced until we come to the correct conclusion: we are responsible for all experiences as co-creators of the said experience, where we can form a different understanding more in line with our soul.

Linear time is a concept whereby time is seen sequentially as a series of events leading toward something: a beginning and an end. Linear time is like an arrow launched from the past, crossing the present and heading for the future. This is a problem for living or being in the moment. This is where we rush to accomplish ego-defined goals, which can drive us through our lifetime. I usually call this playing badminton between your past and the future. This continuing struggle comes at the expense of not paying attention to more significant life signals such as the body, the intuitive mind, and guidance, which only comes in the moment now. Negative emotions from the past or obsessive passions for the future both block intuitive guidance. Guidance is subtle, while emotions carry a lot more energy than intuition, which requires one to be calm and relaxed. This is why meditation and mindfulness are strongly suggested as daily practice.

"Early in the journey, you wonder how long it will take and whether you will make it in this lifetime. Later you will see that where you are going is HERE and you will arrive NOW...so you stop asking."

– Ram Dass, Be Here Now

To that point, Michael Talbot, in his book "Holographic Mind," presented a study where two neurophysiologists measured the time it took for a touch stimulus to register on a patient's skin to reach the brain as an electrical signal. The study requires patients to push a button when they become aware of being touched. They found that the brain registered the stimulus 0.0001 seconds after it occurred, and the patient pressed the button 0.1 seconds after the stimulus was applied. The patient didn't report being conscious of the stimulus or pressing the button for almost 0.05 seconds. This indicates that the unconscious mind was responsible for the conscious mind pushing the button. The delusion is that the conscious mind is in control of the action. This is how intuition and spiritual guidance work. Spiritual suggestions are always at work, whether we recognize them or not.

"Spiritual learning does not occur in a linear progression like logic. It is more that familiarity with spiritual principles and disciplines opens awareness and self-realization. Nothing "new" is learned; instead, what already exists presents itself as completely obvious."

– Dr. David Hawkins

We are much too driven by memories, needs, desires, appetites, and emotions at the ego level, and attempts to continue these choices can cost us dearly in our lives. They separate us from our soul's purpose, self-realization, or Divine Consciousness. When dealing with the conscious mind, we must remember to see things as they are, stay in the moment, and accept them. The Universe is perfect, and nothing we do can or needs to change that.

"Self-realization is knowing in all parts of body, mind, and soul that you are now in possession of the kingdom of God; that you do not have to pray that it come to you; that God's omnipresence is your omnipresence; and that all that you need to do is improve your knowing."

-Paramahansa Yogananda

Why the Universe is Viewed as Perfect

The universe works under steady and transparent laws like gravity, electromagnetism, and thermodynamics. These rules control everything, from galaxy movement to atom behavior, showing a basic order. Even what seems chaotic still has some patterns. Everything in the universe is connected, creating a system in which each part aids and affects the whole. This interconnection shows a form of unity and balance. Life and systems in the universe continually change and adapt. From the birth and death of stars to the evolution of ecosystems, the universe's processes sustain and renew.

The universe runs on time and space scales that usually go beyond human understanding, hinting at more profound wisdom and intelligence. Its vastness and timeless characteristics suggest a form of perfection that exceeds single moments or events. The visible struggles, challenges, or chaos in the universe often create chances for growth, learning, and change. These differences underscore the active and meaningful nature of existence.

"Life is a series of natural and spontaneous changes. Don't resist them; that only creates sorrow. Let reality be reality. Let things flow naturally forward in whatever way they like."

– Lao Tzu

One of my favorite country songs is Garth Brooks's "Dance." The line that says it all is, *"If I would have skipped the pain, I would have missed the dance."* How often has a traumatic experience turned into the best thing ever in your life? We are incapable or conscious of all that spirit can bring into our lives—one moment at a time. And the spirit can give us a far greater life than you can imagine—one moment at a time.

"Everything has already been decided. It was known long ago what each person would be. So there's no use arguing with God about your destiny."

– Ecclesiastes 6:10

I sometimes use this quote to help people see that their struggle has a gift to offer. When we accept what life has to give us, we grow. The collective experiences of a lifetime will eventually come together to bring us closer to Universal Consciousness.

"Don't let those things which may not in the present be understood weary the soul, but know that sometime, somewhere you, will understand."

– Edgar Cayce, Reading 5369-2

Living in Now

"Take care of each moment, and you take care of all time."

– Buddha

Have you ever watched a Hummingbird Feed? You can't help but feel awe, a moment where you pause. That is living in the moment. Why would we not want to pay that much attention to everything life offers? People, nature, the beauty of the planet, and the universe can give us pause. But the ego doesn't allow pause for long before it jumps in to dominate our thoughts and regain control. Regrets about the past or fears about the future can take over our minds, making it hard to enjoy the present. We can have anxieties when sitting at a stoplight. The challenge is to be an observer of life and our thoughts.

"Stop thinking and end your problems."

– Lao Tzu

We are the evaluators of what we think. We decide if what the ego-thinking mind is saying is valuable or not. Pay attention to the physical senses as you do things. Getting used to living in the present moment could become something you do every day. Even so, I try to get some anxiety-conflicted clients to start living today. That alone will help us focus on what's in front of us instead of comparing what was to what's happening right now. Creativity is NOW!

"Man has no choice other than to use his creative power. His thought will always be creative, whether he knows it or not. The creativity of man's thought has nothing to do with his will or belief; it is here just as nature is. It is the use of a creative power that man has control over, not the thing itself."

– Ernest Holmes, The Science of Mind

Man's most extraordinary power is visualization. When we know what we desire, we must visualize ourselves receiving it with faith and intensity. Creating the future must be visualized with a feeling of attainment. We are always in the now when we visualize our excitement. Excitement comes from desire, along with inner and outer sight.

"Realize deeply that the present moment is all you ever have. Make the Now the primary focus of your life."

– Eckhart Tolle

Being present means being fully aware of and active in the here and now without the past or future getting in the way. The first way to evaluate our thoughts is to understand how our body responds to any moment. If an idea doesn't feel good, reject it. This can help us be in the present, calm our minds, and bring our awareness to the Now. Remember, the ego loves to connect with the past and imagine what will happen in the future, which causes unnecessary pain by focusing on worries and regrets. We can learn to notice our thoughts without getting caught up in them. We can also understand that we are not our thoughts but the awareness that supports them.

"I didn't arrive at my understanding of the fundamental laws of the universe through my rational mind."

– Albert Einstein

I teach clients that my favorite way to stop overthinking or just thinking, in general, is to pick a spot and focus on it for ten to twenty seconds. You are not thinking because the conscious mind can only do one thing at a time. If you want to change the moment's reality, focus on breathing. Close your eyes. Breathe in through the nose to the count of five and exhale through the mouth to the count of eight. Pay attention to the temperature of the air and the rhythm of your breathing for thirty seconds. When you open your eyes, you will pause as you readjust to a new reality.

"You should sit in meditation for twenty minutes every day – unless you're too busy. Then you should sit for an hour."

– Zen proverb

Some could be better meditators. I am one of them. I have found several other ways the Spirit speaks to me. When I'm listening to music, in the shower, even when I ask a question out loud. People have different ways of communicating with their higher selves. Different minds have various modes of communication with an inner knowing or psychic ability. Yet we are all endowed with an intuitive knowing. Listening to this guidance can profoundly affect your life and be at peace with everyday activities.

"Intuition (is) perception via the unconscious"

– Carl Jung

Intuition or a gut feeling is an understanding or knowing of a situation without specific data or evidence at the time; analytic reasoning is not part of the intuitive process. Instinct is an innate, hardwired tendency. For example, humans have biological, hardwired instincts for survival and reproduction. Intuition is the ability to acquire knowledge without inference or reason. The word intuition comes from the Latin 'intueri,' often roughly translated as 'to look inside' or 'to contemplate.'

"Intuition is the strength of the soul...we are wired through our intuition."

– Caroline Myss, Medical Intuitive

Forward Focused is Our Power

In the Aquarian age, where man's brotherhood is the hallmark, service to others and the world will become far more critical as we develop a consciousness of service to others and self-forgetfulness. When we use our creativity and service for the betterment of others and the world, we become ever more infused with Divine Consciousness. This is the Aquarian Age, where the principles of freedom and equality are honored above all else.

"Truly, the greatest form of world service is to live life in conformity with spiritual truth, for then every service you provide will affect the destiny of humankind."

– John Randolph Price, Angels Within Us

Using the Mind

The subconscious mind is a positive imagining unit for the future. It precedes a desire by visualizing what you do want. The job then becomes the step-by-step process of action toward making it happen. Since the subconscious is responsible for ninety-five percent of our reality, according to neuroscience, it should become our dominant way of using our most powerful mind.

"When you see a thing clearly in your mind, your creative "success mechanism" within you takes over and does the job much better than you could do it by conscious effort or willpower."

– Maxwell Maltz, MD. The New Psycho-Cybernetics

Your starting point begins in the now, stimulated by desire. Inner and outer sight activates emotion, shaping and attracting your vision and triggering physical expression. Staying in the moment allows the soul to command the emotional body, where excitement toward achievement is necessary. The final act is to let go of expectation, the souls in charge.

"To carry on a successful business, a man must have imagination. He must see things as in a vision, a dream of the whole thing."

– Charles M. Schwab, Industrialist

Visualization and imagery should focus on achieving a desired goal. Hold the vision in mind while intensifying the details for ninety seconds, then take the first action toward fulfillment. This stimulates the brain, where vision draws new neuropathways that send electrical impulses throughout the body and the auric field. The subconscious will intensify your vibration to attract, repulse, and adhere while providing cohesion and eventual manifestation.

"Create a mental blueprint of the object you wish to produce. In detailed picture form, it should be a definite size, proportion, substance, density, color, and quality. Create a mental matrix of the desired object, then determine where it manifests. If you don't know the atomic pattern, call on the Divine Intelligence within your Higher Mind to register the pattern for you from the Universal Intelligence and impress it upon your memory body and your mind."

– St. Germain, Alchemy, by Clara Barton

The Challenge

Life is like photography...we are developed from negatives.

Worry is the dark room where negatives are developed.

Beautiful pictures are developed from negatives in a dark room...so if you see darkness in your life, be reassured that a beautiful picture is being prepared.

Life is like a camera. Focus on what's important, capture the good times, develop from the negatives, and take another shot if things don't work out.

– Unknown

Our capacity for past and future thinking is connected to mental time travel. Although we try to focus on the present, our brains can travel back to consider past occurrences and picture future opportunities. We often need help to fully utilize this remarkable ability. We usually concentrate on short-term rewards and expenses rather than using mental time travel to arrange and prepare for the future; we favor quick gratification over long-term benefits.

231

"Your beliefs become your thoughts, thoughts become your words, your words become your actions, your actions become your habits, your habits become your values, and your values become your destiny."

– Mahatma Gandhi

Valuing the present over the future will help us make decisions that might hurt others and ourselves. There can be significant consequences for short-sightedness. For example, we might refrain from participating in bad habits like binge eating or skipping workouts without thinking about the long-term effects on our health. Analogously, we can overlook environmental issues, including climate change, if the effects seem far-off and abstract. Ignoring the future runs the danger of creating problems that would become progressively more work to address over time.

"He who values the world as his own body can be entrusted with the empire."

– Lao Tzu

One main reason we neglect to prioritize the future is cognitive biases, which shape our decisions. Present bias and hyperbolic discounting lead us to give quick rewards and top priority over future benefits. Moreover, our brains would rather depend on well-established routines and habits than actively assess fresh choices. To overcome these biases, we must consciously consider the future of our decisions and possible consequences.

"Anytime you're gonna grow, you're gonna lose something. You're losing what you're hanging onto to keep safe. You're losing habits that you're comfortable with, you're losing familiarity."

– James Hillman, Psychologist

Finally, exercising free will requires active future navigation. By assuming our destiny and making purposeful future decisions, we might design the life we wish for. This calls for a commitment to lifelong learning and development and an openness to change and adaptation. By engaging in mental time travel and prospecting, we may overcome the constraints of our past experiences and create a better future for ourselves and others.

"We are not permitted to choose the frame of our destiny. But what we put into it is ours."

– Dag Hammarskjold

Mindfulness is sometimes seen as antagonistic to reaching goals, yet it can help us achieve our objectives and enjoy life more. Being attentive helps us to appreciate daily tasks, including apparently boring ones like housekeeping.

The following are 11 easy techniques to include mindfulness in a busy life:

Stressing one activity will help you avoid multitasking. This enables us to be entirely present and value our work more.

When working on a project, take your time and maintain focused and deliberate motions. This helps us to appreciate the process and concentrate on the work.

Concentrate on what matters. This helps us to focus on a small number of tasks and complete them more slowly and carefully.

Space between items on your itinerary can help avoid feeling rushed and explain unexpected delays.

Spend at least five minutes daily not doing anything. Spend time each day sitting silently, focusing on your breathing, and noticing your surroundings and thoughts.

Stop obsessing over the future. Become more aware of your ideas and note when worrying about the future. Practice returning to the present.

Focus on the person you are talking with and listen to them instead of stressing about what you will say next.

Eat slowly and savor meals instead of rushing through them.

Approach all activities with a calm and deliberate delight, concentrating on the sights and sounds around you, therefore savoring your existence.

Focusing your whole mind on the activity and doing it wholly and gently will help you make cleaning and cooking a meditation.

The most crucial thing is to use mindfulness, even if you feel annoyed constantly. Breathe deeply, imagine a white light entering the top of your head and going straight down your spine, center yourself, and relax. Your reality has changed.

Cultivating your Spirit

Living in the present helps you connect with your higher self and prevents you from focusing on past mistakes or future anxieties. This enables you to communicate with your spirit and have a more purposeful and fulfilling life. When you are future-focused, you are distracted from fears and anxieties, which starve your energy and creativity. Now, you can find joy, peace, and a genuine connection with your Spirit.

"It is through gratitude for the present moment that the spiritual dimension of life opens up."

-Eckhart Tolle

Surround yourself with good energy. Use incense or candles to enliven the sense of smell or flowers to lift your mood. I recommend that some clients put a small water fountain in their home or environment for a sound that soothes emotions. Your environment should solicit positive emotions like peace, love, and pleasure that uplift you. All this helps strengthen your connection with spirit and deflate the barriers of the ego.

"Archetypes (the deities) are not airy-fairy irrelevant concepts: they are the fundamental dynamics of the conscious mind, hidden in the psychic depths. They are nodal points of psychic energy in every contemporary psyche, impelling us to actions and behaviors and ways of perceiving and evaluating the realities of everyday life in the here and now."

– Eugene Paschal, Ph. L., Jung to Live By

Connecting with your soul also depends on your awareness of deliberate decisions. Accepting accountability for your choices releases the ego's hold and helps you understand your strength. This enables you to live a more authentic, fulfilled life and make decisions following your spirit.

"The supreme state of the soul is to obey even that against which the mind rebels. And the lowest state of the mind is to revolt against that which the soul obeys."

– Kahlil Gibran

Moreover, you should avoid obsessing and allowing negative self-talk. When your mind is in observer mode instead of validating ego ramblings, you think more in line with your spirit. Turn your attention to a task or visualize something you desire. Maybe even daydream about "what ifs." This helps you follow your intuition and make decisions according to your soul since the soul is responsible for the vision.

Finally, connecting with your spirit requires developing humility. Let go of judgment, criticism, and the need to be correct. Adopting humility will help you live more joyfully and peacefully and strengthen your relationship with your spirit and others. There is nothing or no one you need to defend yourself.

"Humility is merely the truthful acknowledgment of the fact that the ego/mind, by its structure and design, is intrinsically incapable of being able to differentiate truth from falsehood (that is, essence from appearance)."

– Dr. David Hawkins, Along the Path to Enlightenment

Chapter 12:
Soul Fusion with All That Is

Tug on anything at all, and you will find it connected to everything else in the rest of the universe.

– John Muir

Like many others, I've always been fascinated by outer space and what lies there. The television show Star Trek was so enthralling that I watched each episode more than three times, analyzing each character until I knew them by heart. The adventures and possibilities captured my imagination, and how we connected and responded to aliens felt terrific, honest, and fantastic about what the galaxy offered. Here, we are transitioning into the Aquarian Age, becoming more aware that extraterrestrial life has been around us all along.

Connection and Synchronicity

Everything is linked and connected, which implies that each person, object, and event is part of a larger whole and that our actions and energies are present. Two systems of thought suggest the connection: the Hologram and the Morphic Field. Each tells of a dynamic healing opportunity that Hypnotists use to explore age, past life regressions, and superconscious healing. The superconscious mind is a state of awareness beyond regular thinking and understanding. It is seen as a higher type of intelligence or spiritual insight that links people to universal truths, shared consciousness, or divine knowledge.

There is much proof and evidence to back up these theories as applications that promote healing. Dolores Cannon is renowned for such work. Ines Simpson, an award-winning Hypnotist, developed "The Simpson Protocol," a process that allows the client's conscious mind to relax and step aside so the Superconscious can work wholly and freely to benefit the client's optimum outcome. She has demonstrated this worldwide. William J. Baldwin pioneered Spirit releasement therapy, integrating various techniques using regression and past-life therapies for healing. Dr. Deepak Chopra succeeded in healing abilities, surpassing the ordinary conscious mind by advocating a connection to the higher consciousness.

Holographic healing is based on the concept that body, mind, soul, and spirit are interconnected like a hologram, where every part reflects the whole. This method views health not just as physical well-being but as an energetic harmony across all levels of existence where each part of the whole contains information about the entire system. This type of healing is a holistic, multi-dimensional approach that works on every level of a person's being. Profound healing can occur by addressing the energetic blueprint, releasing emotional and karmic patterns, and aligning the individual with their higher self. Whether working on physical ailments, emotional wounds, or spiritual growth, this approach promotes profound transformation and a return to balance and harmony.

Working in the morphic field is another concept where invisible, non-physical fields shape not only the development of organisms but also their behaviors, habits, and even societal structures. These fields serve as blueprints or memory fields that guide the evolution and organization of systems, both living and non-living. These fields are not limited to biological organisms but extend to behaviors, thought patterns, cultures, and even inanimate objects. This supports the idea that morphic fields exist for all self-organizing systems, including plants, animals, societies, crystals, and galaxies.

Morphic resonance is the idea that there is a resonance across time and space, allowing patterns from the past to influence the present. This means that once a particular behavior, pattern, or form is established, it becomes easier for similar forms or behaviors to manifest in the future because the information is stored in the morphic field.

I have had direct experience with these two ideas and concepts in my Hypnotherapy practice. Clients recognize issues that last many years of their lives, creating emotional conflicts and doubts about themselves and their lives. Understanding a medical issue from a different perspective can be a first step in healing beliefs that support disharmony and illness. Deepak Chopra wrote extensively about the mental change of perspectives that leads to healing.

"A significant study of four hundred spontaneous remissions of cancer, interpreted by Elmer and Alyce Green of the Menninger Clinic, found that all the patients had only one thing in common: Every person had changed his attitudes before the remission occurred, finding some way to become hopeful, courageous, and positive."

– Quoted from Quantum Healing by Deepak Chopra

The Soul

"Your intuitive system is wired to alert you as soon as you start losing power; you are alerted of the consequences of every choice you make and have made."

– Caroline Myss, Medical Intuitive

Words shape and create our reality. Speaking expresses oneself and creates a vibration and a belief that will manifest in the real world. This concept suggests that the spoken word is helpful for creativity and expression, as our words may bring things into reality.

Every object in the cosmos depends on one another. This belief is that every element links itself to every other and that everything is a part of a greater whole. This relationship is spiritual, energetic, and bodily. It shows that every action, idea, and choice affects the universe.

"In peace, there is no longer any conflict. There is a total absence of negativity and an all-encompassing lovingness experienced as serenity, tranquility, timelessness, completion, fulfillment, stillness, and contentment. There is inner quiet and light, a feeling of oneness, unity, and total freedom. The peace is imperturbable. Actions become effortless, spontaneous, harmonious, and loving in their effect. Our perception of the universe and our relationship to it is shifting. The

240

inner Self prevails. The personal self has been transcended, with all its feelings, beliefs, identities, and concerns. This is the ultimate state sought by all seekers, whether they are religious, humanist, or have no spiritual or philosophical identification at all."

– Dr. David Hawkins, Letting Go

Spiritual development helps our soul guide us toward change and growth. It is the conviction that, on a path of self-discovery and progress, we are spiritual beings rather than just physical entities. This process helps us become more aware of our genuine essence and connectedness to the universe, enabling our unification with the divine.

"Matter is the vehicle for the manifestation of soul on this plane of existence, and soul is the vehicle on a higher plane for the manifestation of spirit, and these three are a trinity synthesized by Life, which pervades all."

– H. P. Blavatsky

According to this view, the universe is an excellent network of mind and energy. Every sector is interrelated, so every action, idea, and decision affects the whole universe. This connectivity spans physical activity and includes spiritual and energetic elements.

Creative energy controls and directs the universe. It is the conviction that this power drives the universe's development and accounts for all creation. This vitality is often called the "Universal Consciousness" or the "Mind of God." The soul is our everlasting, spiritual component that endures bodily death. This holds that the soul is on a road of development and reincarnation into several bodies and experiences to learn and change. Considered the spark of divinity

241

inside each of us, the soul is the part of us connected to the Spirit, the cosmos, and the Universal Consciousness.

Three levels define humans' unique forms of intelligence: subconscious, conscious, and superconscious. The conscious is the part of our mind that we are aware of; the subconscious is the part of our mind that works behind our conscious awareness; and the superconscious is the part of our mind connected to Universal Consciousness. This three-tiered intelligence helps us communicate more profoundly with the cosmos and reach higher degrees of consciousness.

Our thoughts, ideas, and actions define our reality. It is the conviction that our ideas are tangible objects that can appear in the real world, not only abstract ideas. This idea holds that our intents and ideas will design our reality.

"It is the attitude of the mind which draws the karmic cords tightly round the soul. It imprisons the aspirations and binds them with chains of difficulty and obstruction. ...it will be only through a change of mind that the karmic burden will be lifted."

– The Theosophy Society

Creation and author are inseparable. It is the conviction that the divine is not only produced but also a part of the universe. This unity shows that we are not unique from the universe; we are a necessary part of it and a co-creator of our reality.

The Spiritual Blueprint

"Healing in the present moment involves resolving the unfinished business of the past, which continues to influence a person in the present

moment. Past events' residual mental, emotional, physical, and spiritual energy contaminates the present experience. Resolving the removal of burdensome energies is the goal of any healing approach. Then a person can live more fully in the present and fulfill more completely the details of the life plan that was arranged before the present incarnation."

– William J Baldwin, Spirit Releasement Therapy

A Spiritual Blueprint refers to the unique design or plan of an individual's soul, outlining their purpose, lessons, and experiences in this lifetime. It resembles a map of the soul's journey, guiding one's spiritual evolution and growth. Just as a blueprint lays the foundation for a building, a spiritual blueprint provides the framework for a person's life, including the challenges, relationships, and opportunities they encounter.

What Constitutes a Spiritual Blueprint:

- Why are you here? Your spiritual blueprint contains the essence of this purpose, guiding you through experiences that align with your soul's higher mission. This purpose often involves spiritual lessons you are meant to master, such as compassion, self-love, forgiveness, or wisdom.

- Past-life influences and unresolved karma. You carry energetic imprints from previous lives into this one. Perceptions of activities processed in error cause a perspective or judgment that must be corrected.

- Struggles and themes in life, relationships, or reoccurring situations that present themselves until they result in a desire for change and resolution. A new perspective brings about healing in the body, mind, and soul.

- Vital lessons you've chosen to learn in this incarnation are experiences and challenges, often manifesting through any area of life as continuing struggles. These lessons help you evolve spiritually by pushing you to face fears, resolve past traumas, or embrace new levels of awareness.

- Soul Commitments are agreements made before birth with other souls designed to help each other grow and evolve. These commitments determine all romantic, familial, or any challenging relationships meant to assist you in learning particular lessons. Soul commitments are often the foundation for deep connections and intense challenges, as they are set up to help both parties evolve spiritually.

- Unique abilities, talents, and skills are carried into this life. These gifts are related to what you are naturally good at and aligned with your purpose, allowing you to share them to serve others or fulfill your personal and spiritual growth.

- Challenges that trigger growth and transformation can include health issues, financial struggles, complicated relationships, or inner battles like self-doubt or fear. Rather than being seen as a misfortune, these obstacles are part of your soul's plan to accelerate your spiritual development and help you transcend limiting beliefs or patterns by taking responsibility for every creation.

- You always receive guidance and support from Spirit guides, Angels, ancestors, or other spiritual allies. How well you listen to intuition versus reasoning and logic is a matter of trust that may need work. These guides help you stay aligned with your soul's path, offering protection, wisdom, and subtle guidance through dreams, synchronicities, or intuitive nudges. This support may come through divine timing, signs, or the presence of mentors or teachers in your life.

The spiritual blueprint is dynamic, adapting as you make free will choices and grow. It outlines the evolutionary path your soul will take in this lifetime, offering multiple opportunities for expansion, healing, and transcendence. As you evolve spiritually, your blueprint opens to new potentials, deeper awareness, and higher states of consciousness.

"Accidental, odd, randomness is the inability to understand God's plan."

– Robert Edward Grant, Polymath

How to Access and Understand Your Spiritual Blueprint

- Meditation and Reflection: Quieting the mind and focusing on your inner self can help you access your spiritual guidance. Meditation regularly helps you connect with your deeper desires and intentions, providing insights into your purpose and the lessons you need to learn.

- Astrological Insight: Astrology can help you understand elements of your spiritual guidance. The North Node (spiritual growth) shows your purpose and direction, while planets like Saturn (lessons from karma) and Chiron (healing wounds) hint at the challenges you must face.

- Hypnosis and Past-Life Recall: Hypnotherapy and regression methods may help you uncover memories from previous lives or connect with your inner mind to reveal patterns and contracts affecting your present life. This can be significant in understanding why particular challenges or relationships keep repeating.

- Dream Analysis and Intuition: Your spiritual guidance may be shown through symbols, dreams, or intuitive feelings. Noticing recurring dreams, symbols, or instincts can give hints about your soul's journey. Keeping a dream diary and thinking about these experiences can uncover meaningful insights.

- Energy Healing: Practices like Reiki or chakra balancing can help remove energetic barriers and gain a clearer vision of your spiritual path. These healing techniques can show where you might be stuck and how to better align with your soul's wishes.

- Channeling and Spiritual Support: Collaborating with a reliable spiritual teacher, shaman, or psychic can help you gain further insight into your spiritual guidance. These helpers can assist you in connecting with higher knowledge, showing your soul's plan, and clarifying how to proceed in your life's journey.

Living Your Spiritual Blueprint

Once you understand your spiritual blueprint, the next step is to align with it.

This involves:

- Respecting your soul's aim by being true to yourself and heeding your inner voice.

- Address your life lessons and karmic habits with mindfulness and kindness. Understand that every hurdle is a chance to develop.

- Applying your skills and abilities to benefit yourself and others, aligning with what you bring to collective awareness.

- Keeping a spiritual routine that links you to your higher self and soul's direction, letting your life plan unfold according to divine timing.

Your spiritual blueprint is a sacred plan designed by your soul to guide you through life's journey. It contains your purpose, karmic lessons, gifts, and challenges, all essential for your spiritual evolution. Connecting with this blueprint through meditation, astrology, healing, and self-awareness allows you to align with your highest potential and live a life of deep meaning and fulfillment.

Spiritual Enhancement through Hypnosis

Hypnosis is a powerful tool for understanding Spiritual Enhancement and present-life conflicts. During a session, a client experienced a transforming event when she sensed a figure in a white robe say, "I am always with you, my child." This meeting significantly changed her life, showing how hypnosis might link individuals with greater power or consciousness.

Sometimes, hypnosis is mistaken as either a deep state of sleep, unconscious, or a technique for coercing others into performing foolish actions. But people go in and out of hypnosis every day. In this natural state, the imaginative, intuitive subconscious mind becomes more alert while the critical, analytical conscious mind rests.

People can relax upward into a higher brainwave state called Delta, which offers more possibility for hypnosis than downward relaxation. Everyone has the potential to reach a Delta state of consciousness; hypnotists assist individuals in achieving it, promoting significant healing and spiritual development opportunities.

Deep hypnosis can facilitate clients to the highest self-awareness, bypassing identity and linking with Universal Consciousness, where merging can heal instantaneously. Achieving this state aligns with perfection, where all imbalance is cured. This level of consciousness can encourage spiritual development and insight into demanding challenges, including physical illness and recovery. Higher conscious experience lets people explore new dimensions connected with their souls. This process can enhance spirituality and identify conflicts that have carried over from other lifetimes. The gift of spending time in the Light is priceless. Everyone can achieve higher degrees of consciousness and connect with their spiritual self. Hypnosis can be a valuable tool for spiritual development and advancement.

Soul Fusion Healing: Astrological Analysis-The Universe Speaks

I combined the works of several pioneers and my lifelong pursuits in metaphysics and Astrology to formulate Soul Fusion Healing. A powerful, integrative concept and technique that merges astrology, hypnosis, regression, holographic, and morphic field healing. It guides

248

clients to a connection with the superconscious mind that can bring about profound healing and spiritual transformation. An Astrological chart analysis begins by interpreting a client's natal chart. The Astrology map is a blueprint, revealing karmic patterns, life purpose, emotional wounds, and soul lessons. Astrology provides the map of the soul's journey, showing the critical karmic patterns supporting soul evolution.

"The horoscope for each moment is a set of instructions showing how planetary energies should be used to the best advantage, enabling us to work with them consciously. For every forecast we make, we should attempt to make the cosmic instructions more self-evident so that we can then respond appropriately. "

– Dane Rudhyar, Author: Transpersonal Astrology

Isn't having a five-thousand-year-old art science that symbolizes the universe and changes wonderful? Astrologers call this change evolution. My lifetime of living and observing this beautiful map leaves me with the definition I like the most:

Astrology is an organized system of measuring the universe's bodies that defines the assertion of those bodies, a force of natural energy onto all matter, whereby a language is used to describe the effect of that assertion onto all nature. A forecast of natural phenomena occurs as the universe evolves in a predictable path. Through observation/correlation, understanding the phenomenal influence defines a subjective perspective of the impact on life and human activity.

There are many different Astrological modalities, styles, uses, and as many ways of interpretation as you might imagine. Most are very good, and some are cartoonish and sensational. My preferred interpretation follows my spiritual aspirations and what I call Therapeutic Astrology. This form of astrology focuses on personal healing, growth, and emotional well-being. It uses astrological insights to understand underlying psychological patterns, karmic influences, and energetic imbalances. Therapeutic astrology aims to help individuals navigate life's challenges and release limiting behaviors and beliefs while fostering self-awareness and personal empowerment.

This type of interpretation uses birth charts, transits, phases, planetary alignments, and other tools with psychological, spiritual, and other holistic healing practices. It allows for deeper self-understanding by highlighting the spiritual and emotional influences in one's life journey. It offers guidance, perception change, emotional healing, and inner balance.

"We are affected by planetary vibrations (transits of planets) during our lifetimes because we have attuned ourselves to them during sojourns in those environments."

– Margaret H. Gammons, Astrology: and the Edgar Cayce Readings

Everyone's chart, or what I call a map, has several symbolic signatures. Just like people are unique, each map is unique. The representation of energy in a chart allows free will to rein over how energy is used. It's an individual choice. Conflict comes when we don't use pure energy in harmony with ourselves, others, and universal laws. Observing thousands and thousands of maps, including my own, and understanding each person's journey is fascinating. Yet, seeing the energy of change and transformation with an ability to evolve with the desire and power to do so is a recognition of the "source of all" at work in our individual lives.

The symbolism of the Soul is represented on each map and points to the journey to becoming a purer spiritual self, creating joy and harmony in our lives. We are Light beings who experience a physical Universe. The egos and personalities of the journey are easily explored versus the Soul's desire to attune with the higher Self. Astrologers can explore the residues of multiple lifetimes or experiences where we have come to believe in the errors of our interpretation of life. These are called karmic influences. Interpretative errors are exposed through the conflicts we all experience within our relationships. We have relationships with ourselves and our body, indicating our balance or imbalance, harmony or disharmony, and wellness or illness.

The concept of Soul Fusion begins with an understanding of the blueprint of our life and its challenges, along with positive qualities and creativity. Our guidance from Spirit is always available, and understanding how we approach and use that intuitive voice can be highly important in our decision-making. Readings that offer a more harmonious choice of using energy can and have been highly healing. Changing beliefs change realities, healing our conflicts and our bodies, which hold the conflicts inside, causing disharmony and often illness.

A Therapeutic Astrology evaluation begins with how our past affects our choices of the ego/personality and where a Spiritual path can offer us our greatest reward. A client's clear understanding of how that energy has worked throughout life can determine an area of transformation, steering us closer to a more significant path.

Very few can control the mind that takes us back to the past, where our experience can be fraught with challenge and pain. Evaluating emotional memories can have devastating consequences until we recognize them as experiences that teach us the error in our perspectives and perceptions. Emotional healing comes from the desire to change beliefs and forgive ourselves and others for the conflicts incurred.

There are always challenges and tests at varying degrees for the realities we create. Knowing and understanding these areas where the experiences occur helps us examine the beliefs we use to construct our lives. The weak link in the chain of our beliefs is constantly exposed in various ways. From emotional pain to physical illness, there is always a belief that supports the problems. It is much easier to fix and heal a problem coming to our conscious awareness.

Everybody knows their Sun sign. However, only some people understand the significance of solar power. The idea of our journey is that we are becoming more like our sun sign than the moon sign, representing our emotions and personality developed from the accumulation of multiple lifetimes of experience. The sun represents our vitality in life and our creativity. The moon represents the past. By using solar energy throughout our lives, we become more like our sun sign as we are always in a state of becoming.

Finally, an astronomy reading starts the Soul Fusion process, defining a blueprint of life that is laid out before us. It gives meaning and understanding to the most significant question I am asked. "What is my purpose?" Astrology helps us define that sufficiently with a discussion that will resonate after a reasonable interpretation. When we believe in our purpose, creativity will follow. This step sets the foundation by bringing awareness to the soul's journey and identifying specific areas where healing is needed.

The second step in Soul Fusion Healing is the Hypnosis phase. Hypnosis bypasses the critical analytical mind to allow the subconscious to become proactive in evaluating the circumstances of our lives. I have spoken in earlier chapters about the power available to us through communication with the subconscious. Whether for addiction, pain, or trauma, Hypnosis uses varying degrees of depth to address conflicts. If the desire is to gain a spiritual perspective, Hypnosis can go deeper into the powerful mind to present a unique understanding.

Hypnosis for Deep Connection

The first step is to guide the client into a deeply relaxed state using hypnosis. Use techniques such as progressive muscle relaxation or visualizations that calm the mind and body. As the client enters a trance state, the conscious mind quiets, allowing access to the subconscious and superconscious realms.

Once a client is in a comfortable hypnotic state, I establish communication. Being able to talk with a client for instructions given and feedback on the guided experiences allows for an uninhibited journey. My first guidance is for clients to experience their energy field in a magic mirror. I advise scanning their body's energy field for colors in the auric field front and back. I then have them scan for impurities or a color, usually black, that is out of place on the body. I have found emotional traumas and entities stuck in the field that require healing those emotions or releasing entities that don't belong. The client often made a prior contract to allow them to remain in the energy field.

In all hypnotic engagements, I maintain several Divine presences that can assist in healing and disengagement of attachments. Once the client agrees to release the emotional impact on the body or the release of attachments, my next step is having them journey into the Light. A journey into the light can profoundly affect a person's life. There are usually deep feelings of unconditional love. A client can receive higher guidance on predetermined questions and even guidance on actions needed by the client going forward. I have heard some fantastic advice from and for clients. There are many places to go in the light. You can travel into a regression, move into time between lives, or get advice for the upcoming lifetime. Hypnosis opens the door to deep subconscious healing, allowing access to past-life and soul-level memories. I prefer to start regression sessions once a client has processed the first two steps of Soul Fusion Healing.

Soul Fusion Healing: Regression

Incorporating regression can deepen healing by accessing subconscious memories and releasing karmic patterns that block spiritual growth. The subconscious will typically go to a lifetime relevant to the current life and the client's most profound questions. The subconscious protection will never show something the conscious mind can't handle. Processing a lifetime can involve several significant events. Once completed, I like to go to the last day of life and process the death experience. After the death experience, it is vital to process how the lifetime is viewed. There are several options for processing the death, feelings, emotions, and especially beliefs. Questions about the people and events experienced can be analyzed for possible carryover themes into the next life.

The client is then advised to separate from the body before going into the White Light, where a different analysis can be given. This is always very kind and loving. From this perspective, the lifetime in question offers a spiritual theme that differs from ego/personality. States of higher consciousness can become resources for more profound healing. At any time, a Divine Being can be called in to assist in healing.

Before moving on, many other lives and Universal experiences can be explored. Soul fragments, subpersonalities, altered personalities, and retrieval of lost parts and fragments can all be examined. I have processed numerous lifetimes with clients, each with deep questions for Spirit. After the regressions, I like to go to the client's planning period before the current life. One meets teachers and guides while receiving a plan and commitment to accomplish goals for the coming life. I have always found it fascinating to see the guidance in alignment with the astrology chart.

Sometimes, imagining a future event using the old theme or pattern can be appropriate. Visualizing themselves in a future where the client is healed has a profound impact and a new perspective on life, and it facilitates the steps used to heal current conflicts.

Preparing the Client

- Initial Meeting: Discuss the client's emotional, spiritual, or health worries and determine what issues they want to focus on. This helps tailor the regression to the client's needs.

- Set Goals: Ask the client to decide what they want to let go of or learn during the regression. This helps direct their subconscious mind.

- Getting to a Calm State: Calm the body and mind. Once you reach a relaxed state, guidance or suggestions may occur for various issues.

- Deep Relaxation Methods: Use hypnosis to reach a deep state of relaxation. At this point, visualization and connection become possible, avoiding conscious thoughts. NLP techniques may be used to access the subconscious mind directly. Visualization is critical here.

- Magic Mirror—Into the Light: Looking into the aura or energy field can show where negative energy is stored in the body. Into the Light offers a message from a higher consciousness.

- Emotional Freedom Technique (EFT): Sometimes, individuals or their egos block the experience, and EFT helps clients go deeper and reach a higher level of awareness more quickly.

- Past Life Exploration: Guide the client to explore memories from past lives. Focus on uncovering commitments, karmic issues, or traumas that affect their current life and spiritual growth.

- Soul Part Recovery: Use regression methods to reconnect with lost parts of the soul due to trauma or past experiences. Integrate these parts back into the client for a complete self.

- Childhood Healing: Discuss moments in their childhood that may have led to limiting beliefs or emotional issues. Through understanding conversation, help them heal and move past these experiences.

Soul Fusion Healing: Accessing the Superconscious Mind

"Oriental teachers taught that just as there was a sub-consciousness below the ordinary plane of consciousness, so was there a super-consciousness above the ordinary plane. From the one emerged the things that had been deposited there by race inheritance, suggestion,

memory, etc., while from the other came things that had never been placed there by either race experience or individual experience but which were superimposed from higher regions of the soul."

— William Atkins

At this level of Hypnosis, the conscious mind is wholly bypassed as we set up what we call ideomotor response. This sets up finger signals of yes or no responses where the Hypnotist is in control of asking the relevant questions to the Superconscious Mind.

With the client in a deep trance, they are guided toward the superconscious mind through gentle guidance; we help them connect to their higher self, the purest and most elevated form of their soul essence. Revelations about an illness or disease and its relevance to the chosen life path. At this level, the Superconscious mind can offer guidance or allow healing to occur instantly.

The reigning metaphysical belief is that once the ego identity has passed, there is alignment with Universal Consciousness, where all is perfect, and the body can be realigned. But don't forget that illness and disease have karmic and biological consequences. We must trust that what suits the soul is honored outside the ego/personality. The plan has been put in place for a specific reason: the living and the dying gain positive experiences from the death and dying process.

Superconscious Connection facilitates direct communication with the higher self, offering profound insights, alignment, and the chance to fuse all aspects of the soul into a state of wholeness. In this state, the client can review and realign their soul commitments. They may visualize meeting with their spiritual guides or higher beings who help them understand, renegotiate, or release karmic agreements that no longer serve their highest good.

Soul Fusion Healing and Integration

"If the interest is detached from the plane of sense gratification, if there is a constant effort to fix the mind on the attainment of the highest ideal, the result will be that the past Karma will find no basis in which to inhere on the physical plane."

– The Theosophy Society

Clients are encouraged to release any energetic blockages, traumas, or karmic patterns discovered in sessions. Neurolinguistic Programming uses visualizations to help clients see themselves experiencing the changes in their lives. Soul Fusion visualization can guide clients through visualization of their fragmented soul pieces (due to past trauma or karmic lessons) coming back together and fusing into wholeness. This is the Soul Fusion—the integration of all parts of the self into a unified, healed state. Clients are encouraged to feel this wholeness permeating every part of their being. Having the client affirm their new state of being and commit to living from their higher self and soul alignment moving forward. Affirmations could include statements like, "I embrace my soul's purpose with love and courage," or "I release all karmic bonds that no longer serve my highest good."

After a session, clients are encouraged to journal, meditate, or reflect on the astrological insights and healing process. This allows for continued integration of the soul's healing work into daily life. This fusion of techniques allows for profound spiritual transformation, aligning the individual with their higher purpose and promoting profound healing.

Astrology readings can help us track the changing energies in our lives. Energy continuously shifting presents new challenges and opportunities for further healing. Life is constantly changing and evolving. Once Soul Fusion Healing is experienced, the process continues to work towards making better choices in our lives that align with changing energies and circumstances. Integrating the therapies in Soul Fusion Healing facilitates a holistic process that addresses the mind, body, and soul, allowing for profound transformation and Spiritual Alignment.

"...there is little difference if you believe that your present life is caused by incidents in your early infancy or past lives over which you feel you have no control equally. Your present beliefs cause your events, your lives, and your experiences. Change the beliefs, and your life changes."

– Seth channeled by Jane Roberts

Bibliography

Dispenza, J 2017 "Becoming Super Natural" Carlsbad, CA: Hay House

Rudhyar, D 1991 "The Astrology of Personality" Santa, NM: Aurora Press

Hillman, J Ventura, M 1993 "We've Had A Hundred Years of Psychotherapy – And We're Still Getting Worse" NY: Harper Collins

Cousins, N 1979 "Anatomy of An Illness" New York: W.W. Norton

Nakazawa, D 2015 "Childhood Disrupted" New York: Simon & Schuster

Lipton, B 2005 "The Biology of Belief" US: Hay House

Spiegel, H Spiegel, D 1998 "Trance & Treatment" US: Basic Books

Baldwin, W. 1991 "Spirit Releasement Therapy" Terra Alto, WV: Headline Books

Talbot, M 1992 "The Holographic Universe" NY: Harper Collins Publishing

Bandler, R 1985 "Using Your Brain for Change" Moab, UT: Real People Press

Rosen, S 1982 "My Voice Will Go With You" NY: W.W. Norton

Porter, P 1994 "Psycho-Linguistics" Shipman, Va: Positive Changes Dist.

Elman, D 1984 "Hypnotherapy" Glendale, CA: Westwood Publishing

Cannon, D 2011 "The Three Waves of Volunteers and The New Earth Huntsville, Ark: Ozark Mountain Publishing

Praet, D 2012 "Unconscious Branding" NY: St. Martins Press

Quartz, S Sejnowski, I 2002 "Liars, Lovers and Heroes" NY: Harper Collins Pub.

Butler, P 1981 "Talking To Yourself" NY: Harper & Roe Pub

Wise, A 1997 "The High-Performance Mind" NY: Penguin Group

Cannon, W 1932 "The Wisdom of the Body" US: W.W. Norton

Baumann, T 2001 "God at the Speed of Light" Va. Beach, VA: A.R.E. Press

O'Hanlon, B 2009 "A Guide to Trance Land" NY: W.W. Norton

Helmstetter, S 1986 "What to Say When You Talk to Yourself" NY: Simon & Schuster

Fiore, E 2005 "You Have Been Here Before" US: ASC

Mottin, D 2005 "Raising Your Children with Hypnosis" US: ASC

Achterberg, J Dossey, B Kolkmeier, L 1994 "Rituals of Healing" Gaithersburg, MD: Aspen Publishers

Ornstein, R 1972 "The Psychology of Consciousness" NY: Penguin Books

Maltz, M 2001 "The New Psycho-Cybernetics" London, England: Penguin Books

Hawkins, D 2012 "Letting Go" US: Hay House

Krishnamurti, J 1954 "The First & Last Freedom" Ojai, CA: Harper & Row

Hall, M 1965 "Twelve World Teachers" Los Angeles, CA: The Philosophical Research Society

Epstein, M 1995 "Thoughts Without a Thinker" NY: Harper Collins

Johnson, R 1991 "Owning Your Shadow" NY: Harper Collins

McLaren, K 2010 "The Language of Emotions" Canada: Sounds True

Okken, R 2012 "The Liberating Power of Emotions" US: Ozark Mountain Publishing

Ross, E Cheek D 1988 "Mind-Body Therapy" NY: W.W. Norton

Kolk, B 2014 "The Body Keeps the Score" NY: Penguin Books

Tebbetts, C 1977 "Self-Hypnosis" Glendale, CA: Westwood Publishing

Murphy, J 2000 "The Power of the Subconscious Mind" NY: Prentice Hall

Lanza, R Pavsic, M 2020 "The Grand Biocentric Design" Dallas, TX: BenBella Books

Weed, J 1970 "Psychic Energy" West Nyack, NY: Parker Publishing Company

Jensen, M 2011 "Hypnosis Pain Management" Oxford, NY: Oxford University Press Inc.

Bandler, R 2008 "Guide to Trance Formation" Deerfield Beach, Fl: Health Communications Inc.

Hawkins, D 2009 "Healing and Recovery" US: Hay House Inc.

Porter, P 1993 "Awaken the Genius" Va. Beach, VA: ATG Foundation

Chun, M 2006 "Ho'oponopono" US: University of Hawaii

McHugh, G 2010 "The New Regression Therapy" US: Greg McHugh

Rossi, E 1993 "Psychobiology of Mind-Body Healing" NY: W.W. Norton

Atkinson, W 1900 "The Complete Works of William Walker Atkinson: Kindle

Simpson, I Robinson, T 2013 "The Simpson Protocol Instruction Manual" Inner Healing Press Publication

Atkinson, W Three Initiates 1900 "The Kybalion: Hermetic Philosophy & 7 Universal Principles: Paperback 2024

Hickey, I 1992 "Astrology a Cosmic Science" US: CRCS Publications

Singer, M 1975 "Three Essays on Universal Law" Gainesville, FL: Shanti Publications

Green, J 1985 "Pluto: Evolutionary Journey" St. Paul, MN: Llewellyn Publishing